Professor Ian Parker, a significant intellectual, has much to teach us. This remarkably frank memoir – captivatingly written – will provide a very helpful insight into so many aspects of psychoanalysis – both its attractions and, even, its occasional repulsions.

Professor Brett Kahr*, Senior Fellow at the Tavistock Institute of Medical Psychology, London*

Ian Parker's wide-ranging discussion of psychoanalysis in international contexts is dazzling in approach, tonality, and themes and presents readers with a history of the problems of response and change. Parker gives us a new approach to the psychoanalytic field through his longstanding development and this is a major contribution.

Professor Deborah Britzman*, FRSC, York University, Canada*

From his student years, Ian Parker began searching for alternatives to the shortcomings of mainstream psychology, and this book is the riveting story of how he grappled with the complex diversities of psychoanalytic thought, eventually becoming a Lacanian analyst himself. Parker's erudite and pellucid prose makes this essential reading for anyone pondering the persisting potential and possible pitfalls of deploying psychoanalytic narratives, especially in political contexts, as he takes us on rollicking journeys through Brazil, Korea, Russia and Japan, while debating with queer theory, Judaism and Islam along the way.

Professor Lynne Segal*, Birkbeck, author,* Radical Happiness: Moments of Collective Joy

PSYCHOANALYSIS, CLINIC AND CONTEXT

Psychoanalysis is a strange and mysterious practice. In his new book, Ian Parker offers insights into his own experiences, first as trainee then as analyst, and the common assumptions about psychoanalysis that can be so misleading, as well as a map of the key debates in the field today.

Beginning with his own history, at first avoiding psychoanalysis before training as a Lacanian, Parker moves on to explore the wider historical development of clinical practice, making an argument for the importance of language, culture and history in this process. The book offers a commentary on the key schools of thought, and how they manifest in the practice of psychoanalysis in different regions around the world.

Psychoanalysis, Clinic and Context will be of great value to practitioners and social theorists who want to know how psychoanalytic ideas play out in training and the clinic, for trainees and students of psychoanalysis or psychoanalytic psychotherapy, and for the general reader who wants to know what psychoanalysis is and how it works.

Ian Parker is a psychoanalyst in Manchester, UK, Honorary Professorial Research Fellow at the University of Manchester, Secretary of Manchester Psychoanalytic Matrix, and President of the College of Psychoanalysts, UK.

PSYCHOANALYSIS, CLINIC AND CONTEXT

Subjectivity, History and Autobiography

Ian Parker

Routledge
Taylor & Francis Group
LONDON AND NEW YORK

First published 2019
by Routledge
2 Park Square, Milton Park, Abingdon, Oxon OX14 4RN

and by Routledge
52 Vanderbilt Avenue, New York, NY 10017

Routledge is an imprint of the Taylor & Francis Group, an informa business

British Library Cataloguing in Publication Data
A catalogue record for this book is available from the British Library

Library of Congress Cataloging-in-Publication Data
Names: Parker, Ian, 1956- author.
Title: Psychoanalysis, clinic and context : subjectivity, history and autobiography / Ian Parker.
Description: Milton Park, Abingdon, Oxon ; New York, NY : Routledge, 2019. | Includes bibliographical references and index.
Identifiers: LCCN 2018060188 (print) | LCCN 2019003879 (ebook) | ISBN 9780429031991 (Master eBook) | ISBN 9780367144326 (hardback) | ISBN 9780367144333 (pbk.)
Subjects: LCSH: Psychoanalysis.
Classification: LCC RC509 (ebook) | LCC RC509 .P37 2019 (print) | DDC 616.89/17--dc23
LC record available at https://lccn.loc.gov/2018060188

ISBN: 978-0-367-14432-6 (hbk)
ISBN: 978-0-367-14433-3 (pbk)
ISBN: 978-0-429-03199-1 (ebk)

Typeset in Bembo
by Taylor & Francis Books

CONTENTS

INTRODUCTION

Psychoanalysis is not what you think

This book explores the development and present-day practice of psychoanalysis through an autobiographical narrative that illuminates the internal shape of this cultural phenomenon and clinical work. I am part of this story I tell about what I learned and what I do. "Europeans," Peter Høeg tells us in his 1992 thriller, *Miss Smilla's Feeling for Snow*, "need easy explanations; they will always choose a simple lie over a contradictory truth." I hope to do better than that, and go beyond Europe as I tell my story. It will sometimes seem as if psychoanalysis is as grim and ridiculous as we are often told it is, but you will also see something of the liberating ethic of the practice. I trace my journey through psychoanalysis and my work as a Lacanian analyst.

This weird practice, psychoanalysis, is treated here as a series of theoretical frameworks and operations of language. Psychoanalysis is one of the rhetorical disciplines in the human sciences, attending to the speech of the 'analysand' – the psychoanalytic patient – and opening a space in their lives in which they may speak well. Autobiographical narrative is also profoundly rhetorical and contradictory, of course, and so the chapters travel through different versions of psychoanalysis, making an argument for the importance of language, culture and history in its first incarnation in Freud's work and even more so through its later mutations and doctrinal disputes.

Those who are hostile to psychoanalysis often think they know very well what it is they are against. They assemble their arguments from a series of well-worn stereotypes of Freudianism that are usually gathered from films, television and novels, occasionally layered with second-hand accounts that rely on psychology or psychiatry textbooks. An underlying assumption in those muddled accounts is that psychoanalysis claims to know what you think, and resistance to the idea that it is a deep form of mind-reading is often at the core of hostility to it. This book shows why that assumption is wrong, why psychoanalysis is not really about what you think. It is not what you think. It is about something else entirely.

The first part of the book traces some of the very good, understandable reasons why people avoid it, why I avoided it for so long. I then move on to describe some more positive encounters with psychoanalysis, before describing my training as a psychoanalyst, and then some of the attempts by those who are smitten with it to apply it to the world outside the clinic. I finish by looking at some of the real limits of psychoanalytic theory and practice.

Psychoanalysis is a theory of subjectivity, of our lived bodily experience of being human; actually it comprises multiple contradictory theories of subjectivity. That very contradictoriness accords better with the complexity of human relationships than many other frameworks in the human sciences. As a clinical treatment it encompasses forms of experience that go beyond consciously elaborated thought, and it grounds the way we think in something peculiar and disturbing that goes way beyond what we are immediately aware of. Its attention both to the body and the beyond raises the spectres of sexuality and the unconscious, a lethal combination as far as its critics are concerned, and so it is with different popular attempts to sidestep those issues that we begin. This is a personal account, but as we proceed you will see that we also need to ground psychoanalysis itself in history, coming to terms not only with how it began but also with how it might end.

ACKNOWLEDGEMENTS

Thanks to all those who helped me think about how to write this, providing a context for working through some of the ideas and commenting on the way I formulated things. They include participants in the Discourse Unit international network, in Manchester Psychoanalytic Matrix, and in the 2018 Summer School in Comparative Social Science Studies at the University of Oslo. Particular thanks to Artemis Christinaki, Chris Dunker, Maria Melnikova, Carol Owens, David Pavón-Cuéllar, Andrew Samuels, Mike Seltzer, Sabah Siddiqui, Sergey Sirotkin and Bob Young who read the text, confirmed that things were pretty much as I described, were happy enough with the account I gave, or corrected what I said. I could not have written all this without Erica Burman who participated in much of what unfolds here and helped me to think about it, a passionate and sensible presence through these times and in the production of the book. I resisted her insistence that I replace the names of living characters with pseudonyms, though she almost convinced me with the example of a famous novelist who could have been named, she said, 'Ivan Ego'. I cannot pretend that all of this is empirically true. More than I would like, it is confabulation of one kind or another. As Freud pointed out in *The Interpretation of Dreams*, "Thought is, after all, nothing but a substitute for a hallucinatory wish." (All the Sigmund Freud texts I cite in the book are in *The Standard Edition of the Complete Psychological Works of Sigmund Freud*.) Notwithstanding that, you should at least be in a better position when you have read this text to make up your own mind about psychoanalysis in the clinic and in context.

1

SCIENCE

Avoiding analysis of the mind

There are many good reasons to steer clear of psychoanalysis. The first four chapters of this book explore some of those reasons, focusing first on the relationship between psychoanalysis and science. I describe how I was born into the world as a rationalist, taught that there is a sharp moral distinction between science and superstition. Psychology and psychiatry thrive on this opposition, and there is also, at the heart of quasi-scientific attempts to dispatch Freud, a necessary link with political movements, with those that either disparage or value the role of subjectivity in human action. We start at home.

Lies

Middleton was a huge crumbling mansion house on the corner of Plaistow Lane and Freelands Road in south London. In the early 1960s I first heard the word 'psychiatrist' there, and it was meant as a threat. The labyrinthine dusty cellars could be accessed through a door in our ground floor flat, one of four apartments in the house, or through a side door down some steep steps, or by squeezing down through the bars in the window wells in the front garden. The remains of plaster busts and blank-eyed heads and broken noses of Romanesque statues littered the cellar rooms, covered in cobwebs and thick deep dust. You needed some courage to go down there, and fear at what you might find usually drove you back up again.

Upstairs on the first and second floors, with balconies from which to view the back garden, lived Mrs Clement with Peter her young adult, fresh-faced son, someone we kids bothered when he was working on his car in the garage, someone I liked, perhaps wanted to be like. There was another, older couple (with a deaf maid): the Quarrington-Adams, almost as frightening as the ghostly cellar folk. They were, I thought, very rich, at least as close as I came to rich folk. Mrs Quarrington-Adams watched the maid at work while Mr Quarrington-Adams got drunk and sometime exploded in anger, occasionally menacing my stepfather, Hugh, who menaced him back. It was a war of attrition.

Our apartment, if the self-representation of it by Hugh and my mother was to be believed, was the home of reason; flexible rationality incarnate, pitted against the fairy tales told by the Church and against those who believed in malign spirits in the cellar, as well as against the over-weening arrogance of those above us who would impose their will.

I must have been under seven years of age. One day the Quarrington-Adams' maid was pegging out the washing on a line strung across one of the old vegetable patches, now no more than lumpy, muddy plots in the decaying mess that was the right-hand side of the back garden. We played on the lawn to the left, stripped the apple trees at the end, and ranged around the edges of the garden in the undergrowth that ran all around the house. It seemed odd that the Quarrington-Adams should have a maid, one of the signs of their wealth, privilege and power, a sign that they were above us. We kids sometimes targeted her, the maid, usually with suspicious looks, but this time with a lump of earth. I lurked in the bushes that stretched into one of the mud plots, picked up a clod and flung it at the washing before scarpering around to the front of the house to do something else.

I forgot about it in minutes, but Mrs Quarrington-Adams, who had seen this from her balcony, did not. She told my mother. I was not sure whether my mother was actually annoyed at what I had done or felt embarrassed rage at us being wrong-footed in Hugh's righteous war against Mr Quarrington-Adams. Teatime was wretched, and bath time was worse. I was in our cold bathroom, which had a bare window overlooking the side cellar door steps, there with my mother as she berated me and I denied throwing the dirt. The more I denied it, the more vehemently she repeated one of her favourite moral injunctions.

Although one of Hugh's favourites, one that he cheerfully threw out as a farewell, was 'Be good, and if you can't be good, be careful', one of my mother's favourite commands, which she insisted on this time as I lay on my stomach in the shallow bath, was 'Whatever else you do, don't tell lies'. Telling lies was the worst of crimes for her: it compounded and deepened all the others. She knew I was lying, she said, and finally, exasperated, angry, she threw out what I guessed was the most vicious threat she could muster. I guessed it from the context and tone, I was struck by it and remembered it with a stab of terror: "I'll have to take you to a psychiatrist." The threat worked. It didn't make me confess, but it was part of the punishment for the crime, and it continued alongside the demand that I apologise to the Quarrington-Adams, and to their maid.

Many years later, when Middleton had long been demolished to make way for a modern block of flats, my supervisor for psychoanalytic clinical practice, Carol Owens, told me that she had recently seen a new patient, a prospective patient, potentially an analysand. They spoke face-to-face in these preliminary sessions, as you do, and when the patient left she saw Carol's couch at the side of the room in Dublin and commented with a question "Do people lie there?" Laughter. Well, yes, the answer is most of the time they do. Lies are the stuff of psychoanalysis; lies we tell others to impress them, and lies that we tell to ourselves – sometimes to comfort ourselves, to reassure ourselves about how good we are and relieve ourselves of shame; sometimes to accuse ourselves, to torment ourselves about real and imagined crimes for which we should feel guilty.

We are each a tangle of lies, and the truth we speak in psychoanalysis is rare and unexpected. For some forms of psychoanalysis, that kind of truth is empirical truth about the facts of the case – did I or did I not throw the dirt, say – facts that we must learn to fall in line with. However, I have learned that truth is profoundly linked to the nature of history, subjectivity and autobiography; it is about taking responsibility for what we have become and what we want. That peculiar existential truth of the subject, which is the concern of psychoanalysis, is something we will return to later in this book. Most psychiatric and psychological practice, meanwhile, is still precisely concerned with a shallow kind of empirical truth, which it reduces to what the psychiatrist or the psychologist knows about reality. This, notwithstanding the caveats and qualifiers offered by some of their more thoughtful adherents. Psychoanalysis and psychotherapy often fall into the trap of trying to track down that kind of truth too, and that makes their conception of what a lie is quite frightening.

I had no idea what a psychiatrist was at that time. Well, to be more accurate, of course I immediately had an idea of what a psychiatrist *might* be from the way my mother used the word as a threat. I had a representation of 'psychiatrist' in mind that could just as well be interchangeable with 'psychologist', 'psychotherapist' or 'psychoanalyst', grounded in a kind of shared reality, symbolic material that runs alongside and reinforces a realm of empirical facts about these professions, a realm it does not really directly correspond with.

It was not merely that a psychiatrist would make me speak the truth, as an absolutely verifiable account that would fit with what Mrs Quarrington-Adams had already told my parents, but that they would break down my resistance, break through my denials, break in to my mind. As I grew up, the word 'psychiatrist' and the madhouse became more closely linked, as my mother described relatives who had been a bit crazy or neighbours who should, she implied, be locked up.

We moved next door, from 76 to 74a Plaistow Lane when I was seven, and Cyril and Inez moved into our old apartment. These two were, my mother implied, a bit mad. This 'madness' functioned as a term of abuse and was used to describe people my mother found frightening, people like the vagrant, 'Biting Mickey', who, she said, used to come to her house when she was a young girl, ask for a cup of water and take a bite out of the cup. Perhaps it should be noted that Cyril and Inez were Irish and Biting Mickey was too I guessed. That was something I noted but didn't know what to do with, and so filed it away somewhere; it worked then well enough as a stereotype to signal the presence of something mad and bad.

My decision to study psychology in 1975 was surely haunted by the ghostly presence of the psychiatrist. Psychologists find out things about what people do and why they do them, I was told, and it seemed more interesting than the other option I could have chosen, which would be a course focused on the anatomy of the hand in a medical faculty, alongside medical students, among the medics, which is where you would find psychiatrists. Anatomy would have fitted better with the other biological sciences, zoology and botany, I was originally enrolled for – but psychology would work better, I thought, as a diverting, fun topic away from real science. To study psychology at Newcastle University as a third academic subject in the first year of a combined undergraduate degree programme was one way of avoiding psychiatry and yet accompanying it. It was here that I learned that psychiatrists are medically trained, and base their understanding of the mind on medicine, searching for an organic basis for madness. Psychologists, on the other hand are devoted to the empirical study of behaviour and of mental mechanisms, testing out models of the mind in laboratory experiments.

Here were two ways of plumbing reality, describing mental processes, knowing the mind, and intervening to bring it in line with the facts. There was no reason to think that psychoanalysis was not also up to this game, and so it, too, was something to be suspicious of, even if it was scorned by self-styled, supposedly-scientific psychology. Psychoanalysis, we assume, will dig deep into what you think, so that is one reason to avoid it.

Psys

While psychiatry and psychology worked hand-in-hand to find out what really happens, psychoanalysis was viewed by these disciplines as being the stuff of dreams. It tried hard to get to the facts of the matter, but it failed. I might have conceptualised psychoanalysis, then, in this way: psychology was the realm of reason, the middle ground, ground-floor Middleton approach to reality that was in line with the balanced way that my mother and Hugh saw the world; psychiatry was the place of omnipotent knowledge and harsh judgement, the place of a higher order to which you should conform, that knows what's what, and is relayed to us by the Quarrington-Adamses upstairs in times of anger as a fearful threat; psychoanalysis, meanwhile, is down in the cellar with the hobgoblins, delusory fictions in which we should not believe.

Step into this version of the psychoanalytic world and you can then view the upper levels of this old mansion as the place of the superego, our apartment as the site of the ego, and psychoanalysis as id. This was the crude simplified image of psychoanalysis peddled by psychologists, and the first-year psychology course at Newcastle did indeed make it seem like this cellar containing the id was the world of the unconscious. It was a world I knew little of, and of which the psychology I was enrolled to study also really wanted to know nothing.

The psychology textbooks conveyed the same kind of message. The jokey cartoons were designed to show that Freud was a wacky, old guy obsessed with sex; one of the favourites, much repeated, showed figures of naked women curling around his hair and beard. The line was that Freud was someone who wanted to be a psychologist but could never quite get into the discipline. Psychoanalysis was 'pretend psychology' that failed. And it seemed true, that whether you tried to define what people dreamed about or whether you tried to sum up their personalities by the way they were potty-trained, it wasn't something that fitted with what psychologists wanted of their pretend science of behaviour.

Psychology spent a good deal of time lashing out at its enemies, the more formidable or risible pretenders to providing a science of the mind. On the one side was psychiatry, which, because it had its roots in medicine, and because psychiatrists still had to be trained as medics before they specialised as mind doctors, was to be deferred to but quietly mocked. Thomas Szasz's argument that 'mental illness' was a psychiatric myth was wheeled out at the same time that it was made clear that, in practice, psychiatrists were unfortunately above psychologists in the psy-professions' pecking order. Szasz's well-known critique of medical psychiatry in his book, *The Myth of Mental Illness*, was weirdly mirrored by the psychiatrist David Stafford-Clark's account in the profoundly misleading *What Freud Really Said*, where his hero is pressed into the medical frame.

On the other side, the second front psychologists had to defend themselves against, were the untested claims of the psychotherapists and, most amusing, psychoanalysts, who were in alliance with them: that psychology was a kind of therapy that definitely did not work and that defied scientific methodology with its ludicrous fairy tales about the Oedipus complex and the death drive. Some psychiatrists practised as psychoanalysts we were told, more fool them, and Freud himself was a fake psychologist who had long been discredited. It seemed like most of the psychologists we learned about were dead, but Freud was deader than all the rest.

Freud here seemed to be hoist with his own petard. His account of psychoanalysis as a therapy, debunked by psychologists and psychiatrists in randomised controlled trials, which purported to show that people did not get better when measured against scientific criteria, was part of a grander theoretical framework. On the one hand, at a micro level, Freud grounded his claims about the nature of the mind in his neurological training, and his claims about the effectiveness of his early 'cathartic' treatment and then the full-blown 'talking cure' were addressed to the scientific medical community, tailored to their concerns about effectiveness and outcome. On the other hand, at a macro level, Freud saw psychoanalysis as a key player in a third wave of truly civilised medical practice, in which fully scientific reason surpassed the earlier periods of human history – past times bewitched, first of all, by animist assumptions about human beings at the mercy of a mystical nature, and then by various organised religions. Psychoanalysis was to be viewed as a natural science, but the problem was that the sciences of the mind in the twentieth century were setting it tests it could not pass.

The Newcastle University psychology course dispatched Freud in quick order to the realm of the quacks in a lecture that treated him as an amusing diversion, a joke, and as a prime example of outdated fake science. We 'tested' some ideas about the relationship between food intake and reports of dreams in a first-year group experimental practical class report, that is, an issue actually quite peripheral to psychoanalysis, and moved on. I was puzzled, found the lecture good fun, but was left feeling uneasy more by the scientific high ground taken by psychology than the failure of psychoanalysis to jump the hurdles set up for it.

If there was really something wrong with psychoanalysis, that crookedness was surely bound up with the forms of psychology and psychiatry that were happy to judge it. Perhaps there was even a double problem to be faced here. I could see that psychology itself was not at all scientific and its jibes at the shortcomings of its medical rival, psychiatry, were quite hollow. The laboratory experiments we carried out and read about in the journals were clearly parodies of scientific investigation. The experimental 'subjects' were taken out of their real lives and subjected to bizarre situations so that their behaviour could be observed and their responses to tasks measured. The rationale was that this would test hypotheses about the nature of mind, mind in general, but the findings were flimsy and the extrapolations from them absurd. More than that, and here was the other aspect of the problem, our 'subjects' were always second-guessing, reflecting on what the aims of the experiment were. They were not behaving as scientific objects would do, even though the term 'subject' credited them with a kind of agency that was stripped away in the course of the study, reduced them to the status of objects. So, perhaps it was not only that psychology was not a science, but that it should not be a science at all.

If that was the case, if psychology was mistaken in turning human beings into objects and was acting hand-in-hand with psychiatry as a pretend-scientific endeavour to classify and control people, pathologising forms of experience it could not predict and control, then the problem with psychoanalysis might be even deeper than the psychologists made out. Psychiatry most of the time stayed true to the neurological origins of psychoanalysis, treating bad behaviour and anomalous experience as symptoms of underlying disease entities. It was, in its most strictly medical forms, the forms scorned by Thomas Szasz, still materialist, but a twisted kind of materialism that reduced us all to brute matter. Psychology, meanwhile, had broken away from philosophy and attached itself to an image of science, aiming to study different models of the mind that were weirdly disconnected from the body, trapped by a method that was supposed to be based in the natural sciences; materialist maybe, but operating within idealist conceptual schema. Psychology was a child of Descartes, a figure central to the elaboration of a now taken-for-granted split between mind and body in Western and then global culture, and it, psychology, was stuck with a strictly dualist notion of what there was in the world, ontology, and how we should go about knowing more about it, epistemology. The fantasy was that minds joggled around inside our skulls, and that society was no more than a collection of these abstracted minds, mechanisms to be unpicked by scientists, which is what psychologists imagined themselves to be.

Psychoanalysis was the worst of both worlds; it was building on the neurological medical heritage of psychiatry with a complex, contradictory model of mental mechanisms, and wanting to have the status of a respectable psychological theory.

At least, that's the way it seemed from the way it was framed in the psychology textbooks. Psychoanalysis delved deeper than its rivals, but could not come up with robust evidence that would satisfy them, and so it kept digging. And as it did so, it reinforced the very scientific disciplines that shunned it. It bought into the different categories of personality and disorder that psychology and psychiatry traded in, and it subjected people to interpretations based on those kinds of pathologising quasi-scientific descriptions of what was normal and what was not. To jump into psychoanalysis from psychology would be to go from the frying pan into the fire. It was not scientific, and it should not have pretended to be so, so here was a good reason to avoid it. *Enough of that.*

Spies

A surrealist poster print of Salvador Dalí's 'Metamorphosis of a Narcissus' was tacked up over the fireplace in the sitting room of our shared student flat in Benwell, an old shipyard district in Newcastle. A comrade from the Marxist group I had recently joined asked me, when he saw it, why we would have a painting by a fascist on our wall. He was right to ask: Dalí had sided with Franco during the Spanish Civil War, and had sold out quite early on, suffering, and enjoying, the disapproval of his old surrealist comrades who anagrammatised his name as 'Avida Dollars'. This picture, taken alongside the many other tortured scenes of sexual anxiety in different double-imaged dreamscapes painted by Dalí, played with Freudian symbolism. Psychoanalysis was around in many different places, even in Newcastle, and it wasn't confined to debate in the psychology department. It clearly wasn't dead.

My involvement in left-wing politics – one of the reasons I did disastrously in the end-of-year examinations at Newcastle University, and had to leave the city to lick my wounds for two years back at home in south London – also threw me into a search for radical alternatives in and against psychology that brought me face-to-face again and again with psychoanalysis. It was psychology that gripped me at Newcastle University, not because it was so good at accurately picturing what hid inside our heads, but precisely because it was so bad, so wrong, and so powerful. I wanted to switch from the biological sciences that I had originally decided to study to psychology, to find out how it worked from within. If I was going to do that I needed to know what Marxism and other radical movements made of it, what the criticisms were, so I would be better prepared when I resumed my studies. Everywhere I looked, whether it was in the fleeting references to radical psychology in philosophy journals or in Marxist journals such as *Ideology and Consciousness*, which began in 1977, or in discussions of radical therapy as anti-capitalist and anti-sexist liberation, psychoanalysis was on the agenda.

The complaints against Freud in these places were also harsh, harsher if anything than those I'd heard in the Newcastle psychology class, but they had a different direction. Instead of aiming to dispense with Freud and the psychoanalytic tradition altogether, these were excoriating critiques in debates that wanted to reclaim something, find something positive in what Freud said. I began to wonder if they were right; just as there was something potentially liberating in surrealism, as well as something profoundly reactionary among some individuals who were part of that movement, perhaps there was something in psychoanalysis that could be redeemed. It seemed to be the cultural and political debates that were working at the possibly radical edge of psychoanalytic ideas that were most important, however, not its place as a 'treatment'. That separation between culture and the clinic, between political struggle and the treatment of distress, marked a dividing line that I found very useful in making sense of what I was reading.

The Marxist group I was a member of was Trotskyist, and was wracked with many internal squabbles, including bitter disputes about the place of feminism and the argument in 'second-wave' socialist-feminist politics that 'the personal is political'. Here again psychoanalysis had something to say, and those involved in the debates began to read Freud and various 'post-Freudian' writers. These internal arguments chimed with the *Ideology and Consciousness* journal's early issues, which linked psychoanalytic ideas with feminism, with semiotics as a 'science of signs', and with 'structuralist' theories of language, theories that displaced attention from biologically wired-in developmental processes to language and history.

These arguments didn't go down well with some of the male comrades in the group, particularly those in positions of power, who felt threatened by feminism, threatened by different, more democratic and accountable, conceptions of leadership and organisational structure. The counter-attack often came from those who wielded 'science' as the knock-down argument as to why Marxism stood the test of time and psychoanalysis did not; at root, the argument was that Marxism was a science and psychoanalysis was not, still less new forms of psychoanalysis that looked to structuralism or semiotics instead of biology. I wasn't sure whether Marxism as such was really scientific, maybe because I had become a little allergic to these kinds of claims for science as a foolproof world view from my first encounter with academic psychology, and I did take seriously the feminist argument that Marxism needed to learn from different forms of exploitation and oppression.

The kinds of struggles that inspired many Trotskyists in Britain at the time, particularly my own group that had sister-organisations around the world, were the new waves of protest in the late 1960s and early 1970s that also seeded the women's liberation movement and socialist-feminism. One key reference point was the Vietnam War and another was the May 1968 rebellion in Paris and other European cities, which then linked up with similar uprisings outside Europe. Again, Freudian ideas about repression and revolt, about unconscious desire and its cathartic release in the student demonstrations, were potent as signs that revolution was possible and that it was always latent, always possible.

There was another factor to put into the mix, which was that, the more these ideas caught on, the more the groups that relayed them to the masses grew. It wasn't so much that they grew in size, but that the number of groups grew as they purged internal enemies or split and spawned new players in the sectarian swamp that exists in much of far-left politics. Some of the groups, frustrated and angry at this process had a ready explanation, police agents must be at work. Some of the purges were aimed at police agents, some of the purges were probably engineered by police agents, and a conspiratorial mindset took hold in some groups, leading to physical attacks on rival groups that were assumed to be infiltrated and controlled by the capitalist state.

The accusations and rumours probably did more damage than the spies themselves, and the speed and virulence with which suspicion took root did invite some kind of theory of paranoia. Perhaps it was not so much because psychoanalysis was so good at accounting for paranoia – the mainstream Freudian tradition saw it as an expression of repressed homosexuality – but that it keyed into the sensibilities of old activists, who were despairing at what could be done on the left and in the feminist movement, and who were, one by one, deciding to go into therapy, either as clients or to train as therapists, or even as psychoanalysts. The behaviour of some of the male-dominated left groups even made the idea take off in some circles that paranoia was indeed something to do with male bonding and unacknowledged homoerotic feelings that spun out as displaced aggression against rivals.

By the time I started my psychology degree course in Plymouth in 1978 I had become thoroughly socialised into softer cultural quasi-psychoanalytic ways of seeing the world and Marxist politics, still a Trotskyist but with a new Situationist poster pinned up on my bedroom wall; comrades on barricades embraced, and above them was the legend in French, I translate, 'the more I make love the more I want to make revolution, the more I make revolution the more I want to make love'. There was clearly a gap between all this political activity and scientific psychology. But there was also a gap inside the politics, between a romantic image of revolution powered by unconscious desire and a Marxist science of capitalist economics and resistance. Perhaps it was all very well having an alluring idea of what revolution could be, but perhaps unscientific psychoanalysis was also a dead end if you really wanted to know what the fault lines were in a political system, so you could mobilise the working-class to overthrow it. Psychoanalysis was not a science but an ideology, and so here was another reason to avoid it.

So, I suppose what I had learned about Freud so far, from my first encounters with the discipline of psychology and the hostile comments that psychology made about psychoanalysis, didn't inspire confidence in psychoanalysis, but nor did I have much confidence in psychology itself. There was not much more reason to believe psychology's pronouncements about psychoanalysis being unscientific than to believe its own tall tales about politics, its reductive ahistorical stories about individualism and competitiveness. What I learned about Freud from my political comrades was a little more ambivalent, but often just as harsh, condemning psychoanalysis for not really being a science, this when I wasn't sure that Marxism was a science or whether it should be. There were certainly 'scientific' grounds for rejecting psychoanalysis, but those grounds were themselves a bit shaky. I was looking for a link between love and revolution that had something more to say about both than pretend-scientific accounts of human sexuality and the possibilities of changing who we had become.

2

SEX

Avoiding analysis of the body

Here is another reason to avoid psychoanalysis, it seems. It reduces everything to sex, and, in the process of doing that, it reinforces sexist ideas about the nature of femininity, ideas that feminism quite understandably rebels against. In this chapter I describe how existentialism provides another frame for thinking about science, and how it opens the doors to the Frankfurt School, specifically to the work of Erich Fromm, and then, in more explicitly activist vein, to Wilhelm Reich. You will see why I could have even been seen as a Reichian at one point, but one still allergic to biological essentialist and reductionist accounts of sex in clinical psychoanalysis.

Existence

Feminism followed me down to Plymouth, accompanied my political work in the student union, and shadowed my reading of psychology. It was a counterpart to my search for Marxist critiques of psychology, and it warned me off psychoanalysis. Well, it warned me off taking psychoanalysis seriously, while still reminding me to keep an eye on it. Many Marxists, including those attempting to develop a genuinely scientific Marxist psychology hatched in the Soviet Union, wanted to take psychology more seriously than I would have liked. Feminist arguments drew me away from this unthinking worship of science as such, from scientism, into more radical alternative frameworks based within the philosophy that psychology had cut itself off from when it launched itself into the world as a separate discipline in the late nineteenth century. Dialogue between feminism and Marxism in radical philosophy pulled me into existentialism, puzzling about the meaning of life and what it was to be a human being thrown into the world, an approach that was more on the side of the human being than psychology, which seemed to be very much on the side of the world and what it demanded of us.

Existentialism was cool, it connected better with the world of love and revolution than cold scientific method, and it came kitted out in Marxist colours in the work of Jean-Paul Sartre, and with feminist sensibility in the work of Sartre's partner, Simone de Beauvoir. While Sartre railed against capitalism, was active in political campaigns around a number of issues in France, and was arrested in 1968 during the rebellion there, de Beauvoir mobilised young women against the texture of patriarchy, the kind of society that, as Kate Millett told us in her passionately-argued *Sexual Politics*, was based on the rule of men over women and of older men over younger men. When the existentialists talked about existence, they hedged their bets about the existence of the unconscious, but they couldn't let Freud go. In some mysterious way, psychoanalysis of some kind seemed to be part of the existential frame as an alternative to psychology. This psychoanalysis, however, was to be treated as an existential quest, not as a clinical treatment.

Sartre was hostile to attempts by psychoanalysts to impose their interpretations on their patients, as if psychoanalysis was a complete world view, a grid into which the patient had to fit, a grid that would effectively rob them of freedom rather them lead them to decide for themselves. Sartre published a document in *Les Temps Modernes*, for example, that led to the resignation of psychoanalysts from the journal editorial board: 'The Man with a Tape-recorder' as an introduction to a 'Psychoanalytic Dialogue', both reprinted in Sartre's *Between Existentialism and Marxism*, gave voice to a patient confronting his analyst with a series of interpretations, turning the tables in the clinical session. Sartre claims that it was this rebellious act that enabled what he calls 'the irruption of the subject', something more effective, therapeutic and politically progressive than interpretations given by a psychoanalyst.

And, more confusing, what our behaviourist lecturers in Plymouth were describing when they presented psychoanalysis as a psychological model of the mind or behaviour didn't help in reading Freud himself. I could see that he talked about 'instincts' and 'principles of mental functioning', for example, but I couldn't connect the way he described these things with the ages and stages of development and the lists of personality types in the psychology textbooks. In fact, if anything, my experience of trying to find psychological models in Freud's texts was as mystifying as when I had tried to find something like the neat, sharply-drawn images of plants and animals in the textbooks on the slippery slides of indeterminate stuff under the microscope in botany and zoology classes back when I was in Newcastle.

When Freud talked about 'instincts', for example, he described them not as biological imperatives but as 'drives' that were mediated by the experience of the individual and their culture, as existing, he said, on the border of the biological and psychical. More humanistic psychoanalysts, like Bruno Bettelheim, argued that there was systematic mistranslation in the authoritative *Standard Edition of the Complete Psychological Works of Sigmund Freud*. The German term '*Trieb*' was translated into the English edition of Freud's writings as 'instinct', but should actually have been rendered as 'drive'. This made better sense of Freud's comment about a drive's status being on the border of the biological and psychical; if Freud had really wanted to treat these drives as animal instincts, he would have used the German term '*Instinkt*'. Yes, he did sometimes use that term, but puzzled away at it, contrasting it with '*Trieb*', and opening the way for psychoanalysis as a practice of speech grounded in language and culture.

The discipline of psychology was more than happy to work away at Freud's description of the 'mental apparatus' and discredit what Freud said about it, conveniently overlooking the fact that this term mistranslated the German term '*Seele*' or soul. And, as Bettelheim was to point out in one of his last desperate attempts to retrieve the meaning of Freud's own writing before he died, a whole range of terms that seemed compatible with psychology just did not exist in Freud's own writing. Bettelheim had been brought up reading the German original in his own psychoanalytic training and was shocked to discover how badly it was translated into English when he arrived in the United States as a refugee from Nazism. The terms 'ego', 'superego' and 'id', for example, were scientistic neologisms, replacing Freud's own everyday use of the terms 'I', 'above-I' and 'it' (*Ich, Über-ich* and *Es*). What was at stake here was not only the way that psychologists talked about psychoanalysis, but also the way they reinforced a 'psychologised' version of psychoanalysis.

Then, to the rescue came twinkly-eyed, smiley Erich Fromm in a book I mined for an essay on aggression, *The Anatomy of Human Destructiveness*. Fromm had trained as a psychoanalyst, practised as one, and drew on existentialist ideas to reread Freud as a nice humanist instead of as a perverted, reactionary, old sexist. It wasn't that Fromm was explicitly feminist, and he didn't engage with de Beauvoir's arguments set out in her book *The Second Sex* – that 'woman' was configured in patriarchal society as 'other' to the real quintessential human subject, man – but Fromm did provide a way of making sense of what it was to be a human subject as such, spoke to a sense that I had as a man; that while I was told that men were the centre of the world, I felt off-centre most of the time, alienated from it.

The common-sense and psychological reference to 'instincts' to explain aggression would apply just as well to sex, and would turn Freud's apparent obsession with sexuality as being the root of all human action into a symptom of the very world he was describing. Fromm argued that Freud was very good at describing the predicament we found ourselves in as we struggle to find meaning in sets of social relationships that are themselves destructive, but that to understand those social relationships you needed Marx and a theory of exploitation and alienation. In much the same way, Marx was obsessed with the economy precisely because the economy in capitalist society assumed an overarching value here and shaped every aspect of our lives. The problem wasn't that Marxism was reductively economistic but that the world Marx described was. In the process, Fromm aimed to turn both Marxism and psychoanalysis into forms of humanism that might complement each other.

In Fromm's book, to make love and revolution was to construct meanings and relationships that would be more genuinely in tune with what it was to be human, to find ourselves as human beings who were necessarily social beings. The reduction of this revolutionary loving to raw sex was an indication of the depth of alienation that we suffered under capitalism, a world that turned human qualities into commodities and then sold them back to us with the message that we need to consume them as if they were things in order to be happy. Fromm's other books on Marx and Freud and the search for human freedom also connected with other philosophical traditions, including Zen Buddhism, with the message that it was the structure of this peculiar lifeworld that distorted our striving for connection with others.

More than that, there was the unavoidable fact of being human, of being born into bodies as part of the natural world that posed existential questions, that would need to be struggled with during and after any successful revolution against capitalism. Blending Freud with Marx might do justice to the socialist-feminist argument that 'the personal is political', but it should not let us off the hook. By the same token, if men were accorded privileged roles in a capitalist society that was also patriarchal, that did not mean they could simply avoid their responsibility for colluding with this by claiming that society made us who we are and that society must ultimately take the rap. We might experience aggression toward others, for example, but that did not mean that we needed to enact it; even if there were aggressive 'instincts', we could see that there were countless occasions when human beings had chosen not to pretend that they were bound by those instincts, as if they were automatons driven to attack others.

In other words, Fromm still drove home the message that we needed to take responsibility ourselves, each and every one of us, for the way we experienced sex as a driving force in our personal relationships, for the way we bought into the idea that it was the bedrock of existence. Ultimately, for all the softening of Freud's work and the shift of focus from uncomfortable themes of sexuality and the unconscious, Fromm's approach was still deeply psychoanalytic, and it drew me deeper into psychoanalysis. This was psychoanalysis as a diagnosis of culture though, not as treatment of individuals. If sex suffused society, indicating something about the nature of the political and existential questions we faced, this was all the more reason to avoid reducing it, reifying it, making it the hard core of clinical treatment as Freud and his followers still seemed to do.

Despite Fromm's good intentions in wanting to connect the personal and the political, his approach still seemed unbalanced, too focused on personal change. He told us, as did other writers in the Frankfurt School tradition of research that he was associated with, that capitalist society was corrupt and corrupting, that there was something about the scientific Western Enlightenment that inculcated a rationalist instrumental world view and encouraged each individual to replicate that rationalist world view inside their own personality. The Frankfurt School, which was founded as the Institute for Social Research in 1923, provided theoretical resources for rethinking what 'personality' was as something that was always already social.

When leading figures from the School fled to the United States from fascism, they returned to 'personality' as a touchstone of democratic society, but in the early years, when Fromm was involved, it housed a critique of the personality with an eye to social structure and political change. The Freudian name for that rationalist entity in the Standard Edition translation was 'ego'. For all of that, Fromm still appeared to see work on the ego – to make it more flexible and open to the unconscious, more tolerant and accepting of mystical experience even – as work to be carried out by the individuals who harboured it. He called himself a Marxist on occasion, but it was unclear how his talk about Marxism played out in practice.

Energy

There was another figure on the fringes of the Frankfurt School who walked the walk: stocky, scowling Wilhelm Reich. Reich, who was one of Freud's favourites in the early years of the psychoanalytic movement, obtained agreement from the psychoanalytic organisations in central Europe, agreement after a fight and with Freud's help, to make psychoanalytic treatment available to working-class people. But, more important than that, and this is what caught my attention, he made that intervention part of a political campaign, building a political movement. Reich, like Fromm, saw capitalism as deeply destructive of humanity, and he put his energies into overthrowing capitalism, ending that misery at its root. His analysis of the way that capitalist forms of rationality were relayed into the lives of patients focused on the institution of the family. So here, even though Reich could never be suspected of being a feminist, was a critique of society that chimed with what Simone de Beauvoir, for example, had been writing about patriarchy. The family was the key institution that made men and women what they were and made each child follow suit.

The anxiety and suspicion that were inculcated in the personality structure of men, and Reich had most to say about men as the relays of power and as those subject to its immediate effects, entailed the production of a kind of 'character armour' that led them to defend themselves and to strike out at others when under threat. The rationale for reaching out with psychoanalytic treatment to working-class communities while fascism was on the rise in continental Europe, was to provide a space for speaking out and for loosening this character armour, for shaking off the kind of mindset and bodily comportment that was taken on from their 'betters' in the middle classes. It was middle-class individuals, part of what Marxists called the petite bourgeoisie, shop owners and clerks and self-made men, who were most dangerous, crushed in times of economic crisis; they were trapped between the working-class organisations seeking to defend themselves against the onslaught of austerity and unemployment, and the ruling class, the bourgeoisie hanging onto their privileges. In classical Marxist theories of fascism, and for Reich and Fromm, as well as for many of the other writers in the Frankfurt School, it was the middle classes who looked for enemies and looked for a leader to save them.

The danger Reich could see around him was that fascism turned attention away from internal class divisions in society to enemies who were seen as responsible for creating divisions, putative outsiders such as Jews and Gypsies, sexual degenerates, and those who were accused of wasting the resources of the nation (for example, the disabled or mentally ill). Reich responded to the rise of fascism in Germany by trying to explain it as a form of repression, a particularly vicious repressive system that mobilised fear of free open sexuality. This led him to understand the iconography and ideology of fascism as something poisonous that could only be countered by forms of interpretation that were also forms of practical intervention. The aim was sex education and facilitating an experience of sexuality that connected human beings with each other instead of painfully and defensively treating others as objects to be used, and this required campaigning against sexually restrictive laws. This didn't look like a 'psychological' theory in that it wasn't presented as a model of how people should think, a model that could then be tested in a laboratory. One thing that appealed to me was that it seemed to treat psychological theories themselves as obstacles, restrictions on how we think that needed to be questioned and unravelled.

A crucial part of political resistance for Reich, then, was to tackle the different forms of repression that turned each individual into a little fascist, with character armour to match. The force that would break through this repression was twofold: collective political action to overthrow capitalism; and the release of the underlying forces of rebellion that would make that action possible, underlying forces of rebellion that were condensed in sex. Reich's model for revolution was orgasm, the more the better, with open free expression of sexuality the instrument and goal of anti-capitalist action. He took literally Freud's descriptions of the repression of infantile sexuality through the process of child development, and saw sex as the core force that needed to be released if the distorted development of society under capitalism was to be challenged and a new socialist path for development opened up. This psycho-political analysis was the basis for the formation of 'Sex-Pol', the German Society of Proletarian Sexual Politics.

Despite this, and perhaps despite what Reich eventually wrote about biology and 'Orgone' energy, what the early Reich seemed to key into was not so much biological forces, as the experience we had of our sexual lives being suppressed under capitalism, 'repressed', as he would have it, as someone who was turning psychoanalysis into a political analysis of personal life. And whether or not he was a 'biological essentialist' seemed less important than the work he carried out as part of the Sex-Pol movement in Germany in the 1920s, which campaigned for free contraception, sex education and freedom for young people, for what Reich called in the title of one of his pamphlets, 'The Sexual Struggle of Youth', which was reprinted in his book of Sex-Pol writings. A small group of us, mainly psychology students, and mainly concerned with lesbian and gay rights, set up a student union society called 'Sex-Pol', and our main campaign was to get *Gay Times*, the main publication of the gay community, on sale in the student union shop.

There were a number of paradoxes in our Sex-Pol. One was that, while Reich's focus was on the oppressed and repressed working class as a universal collective subject, our group was more a collection of different groups, male gays, lesbians, socialists, who were all quite keen on maintaining their own specific identities. Another was that, while Reich, like much of the psychoanalytic left in Germany, tended to see homosexuality as a symptom of the distortion of natural healthy heterosexuality under capitalism, even as a seedbed of fascism, many of our members were openly gay. We comforted ourselves with the thought that even though Reich himself had some dodgy ideas, he did actually campaign for homosexuality to be legal and saw the re-criminalisation of homosexuality in the Soviet Union under Stalin as an indication that things were going badly wrong there. We knew Reich had been in contact with Trotskyists in Germany, and there was at least one Trotskyist group in Britain, the Chartists, who were republishing and discussing Reich's work.

Maybe we were non-biologically-essentialist Reichians, unsure about whether there really was this 'energy' inside all of us that needed to be released, but happy to link love and revolution as if it did. Anyway, I did for a while think of myself as being a Reichian and enthusiastically read – as a third parallel track of study alongside the psychology curriculum and flow of Marxist tracts – Reich's work, and also read about him. I learned about his life-journey from being a psychoanalyst to being outcast and paranoid, expelled from the Communist Party for being a psychoanalyst and from Freud's International Psychoanalytical Association for being a communist in the 1930s. His later bizarre theories about 'Orgone energy' I took as expressions of this exclusion and suspicion, of isolation and imprisonment, which included his books being burnt in Germany, Russia and the United States (where he died) – persecution enough to drive anyone mad.

We talked a lot about sex, and maybe that was more important to us than actually engaging in it. I have to say that, rational soul that I was, talking about sex was a lot safer than the prospect of completely losing myself in the drives, getting tangled upon the free exchange of bodies we promised everyone else. I could not shake off the feelings of jealousy that were supposed to disappear in the course of our common struggle. Perhaps I expected too much too soon. Far from dissolving, corrosive jealousy and self-possessiveness, both mine and of those close to me, led me to shrink back, enclose myself, protect myself. I wanted Reich's critique to be true, but it was not yet my truth. I didn't know what to do about it. I was confused, what psychoanalysis would term 'ambivalent', torn.

Most of the student union building in Plymouth was underground. Down the stairs we would go, to hector each other in meetings – I found that relatively easy – or to get drunk. That's what I found difficult, and I usually avoided social events, preferring to attend punk concerts in the city on my own – dyed hair but still a dyed-in-the-wool self-contained individual. I would not have gone near an analyst, never have opened up.

We talked about sex in the Sex-Pol meetings and with people we tried to recruit from the proletarians in Plymouth Polytechnic Student Union. For me, Reich was important, but the Sex-Pol society was also important as a gateway into the real hard stuff, class struggle. I was also politically active, one of the few activists in 'Soc-Soc', the union's Socialist Society. Our Sex-Pol intervention was tactical, and psychoanalysis as such was still something to avoid because it would lead to a final reduction to sex, could lead nowhere else. This was reason enough to avoid psychoanalysis as a form of treatment as such.

Discourse

We didn't recruit many new comrades, and what we were doing was viewed as rather weird, a bit 'gay' in the eyes of some of our enemies on the right, but I did learn something from people who didn't want to talk about sex. They weren't all on the right, and they often seemed uncomfortable when we told them that the basis for a free open healthy socialist society was free, open, healthy sex. We had, unbeknownst to ourselves, stepped into the realm of discourse about sex, which was something a bit different from the real thing, but had real effects. I met Michel Foucault down one of the backstreets on the Plymouth harbour front; his book about the history of madness was on display in an artist's studio window, and he accompanied feminism and me, unusual bedfellows those two, during the rest of my time in Plymouth, as I tried to hold true to my Marxism while navigating my way through a psychology degree.

No, I never actually met him, but I tried to find out who he was after reading him, making his work a reference point for my doctoral thesis in Southampton, fascinated as much by the bald, black-leathered image of him as one of the proto-typical 'post-structuralists'; he also appeared in the journal *Ideology and Consciousness* and frightened hard-core Marxists around the place, as the British left tried to grapple with the power of language and 'discourse' in their turn to Eurocommunism in the late 1970s. It was in Southampton, as I worked my way through Foucault's writings on prison regimes and ended up with his description of 'regimes of truth', that I found a way of making sense of this discourse about sex, a discourse I had been avidly promoting in Plymouth, making sense at least of the reactions of those I pushed it to.

Foucault posed the question of sex in a quite different way in the first volume of his *History of Sexuality*. Instead of asking why people don't talk about sex, which begs the usual popular psychoanalytic answer that people will be happier and healthier if they do so, he asked why people talk about sex so much. The idea that sex is at the centre of our being is not so radical, and not so demanding of psychoanalysis, which insists on the role of infantile sexuality and the unconscious, not so radical when you start to notice that the most radical Freudians and post-Freudians are swimming with the main currents of contemporary common sense. We, like those characters, talk about sex all the time, or talk about not talking about it, which pretty well amounts to the same thing, or hint at it, or joke about it, as something deep and hidden and crucially important to us.

In some respects, and he knows this, Foucault repeats some of the Frankfurt School arguments about what key players Theodor Adorno and Max Horkheimer called in the title of their path-setting book 'the dialectic of Enlightenment'. Later writers in later generations of the Frankfurt School would complain that there wasn't much dialectical content to that book, that it was, rather, one long, grim narrative about the way in which we have become separated from nature, and from our human nature, by our obsession with reason. We are haunted by who we are and what we want as human subjects, but repeatedly shut that desire for connection with others out in order to be good, well-behaved individuals, believing ourselves to be 'individuals', isolated and undivided. As forms of surveillance take hold in Western culture with the rise of capitalism, we also learn to perpetually survey ourselves, prisoners of a regime of truth, in which we pretend that we are free in order to better operate in accordance with the rules of reason. Again, here, we are trapped in the separate 'I', the pop-Freudian 'ego'.

Foucault augments this diagnosis of the chains of Enlightenment with a critique of psychoanalysis as a cultural practice that gives a more insidious twist on confession demanded in the Christian church. Not only are we disciplined, and not only do we discipline ourselves, but we revel in that discipline every time we agree to speak to a psy-professional, whether it be a priest or a therapist, about what we desire – as if to speak about that desire will release us from it. The trap, of course, is that the more we speak about what barely conscious wishes inhabit us, the more we imagine that there are deeper and more powerful things to be spoken about behind that first circle of confession. Confession is a spiral that binds us all the more tightly into the belief that there is something unconscious at work within us and that, at its heart, is sex.

There is, Foucault argued, an incitement to talk about sex. We were part of that apparatus of incitement in Sex-Pol, and people were understandably nervous about where it would lead. Instead, Foucault's historical analysis of the emergence of different 'discourses', including discourses about sex and the body, and supposedly abnormal forms of desire such as homosexuality, showed how people seized on such discourses to make sense of who they were, to declare their 'identities' within those discourses. And so Foucault, also, almost, showed us a way out, told us why we should avoid speaking about sex all the time, avoid playing the cultural game of reducing everything to sex, to our sex.

I didn't let go of Erich or Wilhelm when I hitched up with Michel. I was still very much taken with the existentialist vision that Erich Fromm laid out, of the human being torn between their consciously-reflexive free will, the unavoidable nature of that freedom, and the constraints imposed on them by life in the material world, the fact of living inside a body. The human being is hemmed in on both sides, hemmed in by forces of culture and of nature that go beyond them, by what they try to know nothing about, keep at bay, shut out, make unconscious. What Fromm called the 'art of loving' would then encompass the erotic in order to avoid reifying sex. Wilhelm Reich still spoke to the side of me that felt those drives that Freud described as if they really were wired-in instincts, and sought either their release or release from them. We are at the mercy of the natural elements, including those instinctual elements that condition what we want of relationships, and speaking of them as mere drives underestimates their power, working against us or for us. Reich's account of sex eventually saw it as a manifestation of Orgone energy as a life force that enabled him to avoid making sex the bottom line for ever for all human societies.

Now Michel Foucault voiced from a quite different angle the question of how culture shapes and sets the conditions for the way we speak about sex, about what he referred to as the body and its pleasures. Foucault's attention to discourse and the conditions of possibility for sex to be spoken about and experienced in such different ways at different points in history sidestepped, avoided speaking about, sex as such at all. These guys all operated in different ways from within the theoretical tracks of the German Frankfurt School tradition, though Michel, of course, was French, and it was another French guy, Jacques, who I was going to bump into next.

3

SCHISMS

Avoiding analytic politics

As if science and sex weren't treacherous enough territories for psychoanalysis, the field of politics, political intrigues in the institutions that house it, appeared to be worse. I will take you through the arcane worlds of the Imaginary, Symbolic and Real in my first encounters with Lacanian politics, and we will see how the battle over who should be the master and who would be the slaves operates here. There were some crucial and useful ways of conceptualising the place of the human subject in relation to language in these meetings, but the mirror-like personal power plays were very different from politics as I knew it should be, perhaps too close to political manoeuvring on the already existing left, and a warning to keep out.

Symbolic

"You want to be persecuted." That is Malcolm Pines, a psychiatrist and training analyst with the British Psychoanalytical Society, delivering his verdict on Jacques-Alain Miller's talk in Cambridge to followers of Lacan and to some enemies in January 1985. Why am I here and what's going on? We'll get to Miller, symbolic father of one of the main currents of Lacanian psychoanalysis through his World Association of Psychoanalysis, but we need to start with his father-in-law, the main man, Jacques Lacan.

Lacan trained as a psychiatrist before switching to psychoanalysis, which was viewed as a psychiatric speciality in Paris in the 1930s where he underwent his training analysis. A training analyst is a senior-enough figure designated to psychoanalyse candidates aiming to become psychoanalysts themselves, in the French section of the International Psychoanalytical Association, the IPA, which was founded by Freud and colleagues back in 1910. The British Psychoanalytical Society is the British section of the IPA, which is a big deal in the psychoanalytic world. The further back you trace the present-day squabbles between different psychoanalytic institutions, the more tangled things get, and the deeper are the rivalries and scores to be settled. The IPA is at the core of this history – no small beer.

It was the IPA that installed Carl Jung as its first president, and from which Jung had to resign when he broke with Freud, and it had been the IPA that was site of conflict with Alfred Adler, forced out a year before. The IPA looms large in this book because of that organisation's claim, still, to represent all Freudian analysts, to speak for psychoanalysis and to decide who is and who is not really a psychoanalyst. If you are speaking of psychoanalysts, of course, you are also speaking of practising Freudians, and some of the frictions between different groups revolve around who is true to Freud and who really returns to Freud today.

Lacan claimed to return to Freud, a claim that is sometimes glossed as a return to the meaning of Freud, but did so after accumulating some surprising theoretical resources from outside the psychoanalytic tradition. What were seen as conceptual deviations and innovations in treatment led to his exclusion, his 'excommunication' he liked to say, from the IPA. It was a long drawn out process that began in 1953 and culminated in the big split, and the foundation of a new Lacanian school in 1964. He was close to surrealism, friends with Salvador Dalí, whose themes of doubling reflected Lacan's early speculations about the 'mirror-stage' in child development being formative of the ego, and he continued practising as a medical doctor even after he trained as a psychoanalyst, acting as personal physician to Pablo Picasso.

During the 1930s, while he was undergoing his personal analysis, Lacan attended lectures in Paris by the Russian émigré Alexandre Kojève, a Hegelian scholar, from whom he picked up an account of the master-slave dialectic, which also powers the mirror-stage and later relationships. Hegel's philosophical world view had been a fertile resource for many Marxists – Marx himself had grappled with Hegel's idealist approach and turned it around to stand it on its feet in the material world – and Hegel was then attractive to psychoanalytic writers, such as those working in the Frankfurt School. Kojève's lectures on Hegel were also attended by Sartre and other leading French intellectuals, with ideas from them finding their way into existentialism as well as into Lacanian psychoanalysis. Lacan then discovered the linguists Ferdinand de Saussure and Roman Jakobson, a discovery that enabled him to return to Freudian psychoanalysis as a 'talking cure', finally grounding psychoanalysis in language rather than in biology. It is this turn to language in psychoanalysis that made Lacan so intriguing as an alternative to biological psychiatry and normative psychology; a turn to language was something I could appreciate while still trying to avoid the psychoanalytic aspect of his argument. You might think that is impossible. It was.

For Lacan, especially in the key middle period of his work, we are creatures of language, of the Symbolic order: 'The unconscious is structured like a language' – you can see structuralist ideas at work in that claim – and 'the unconscious is the discourse of the Other', a gnomic statement that carries the traces of Hegel and Kojève. And there is something of the spirit of surrealism in all this that gives to

Lacan's writing and public seminars a hallucinatory quality. If nothing else, he is true to the Frankfurt School theorist Theodor Adorno's comment that in psychoanalysis nothing is true except the exaggerations. In Lacan's work, these exaggerations are stretched and wound around each other so that reading him is sometimes very difficult. It is a reputation for opacity that has been defended by the French Marxist Louis Althusser, for example, in the claim that in Lacan's writing you find something of the logic of the unconscious. Here was a Marxist using Lacan to understand the grip of ideology, for me another plus.

I couldn't understand Lacan. You can't blame me. But the term 'discourse', here shadowed by surrealist and existentialist motifs, pulled me closer to him. I assumed that there was some kinship between Lacan and Foucault, that the discourse Lacan was concerned with in psychoanalytic theory must also, in some sense, be the discourse that Foucault analysed in his historical studies of discipline and confession. Jacques Derrida was the third man here, deconstructing texts, including psychoanalytic ones. The link between the three was reinforced by the label 'post-structuralist' and by the debates over this supposed post-structuralism in the English and Philosophy departments at the University of Southampton. The Department of Psychology, where I was registered to do my PhD, wanted nothing to do with that because psychoanalysis was unscientific, and so the Lacan *Écrits* reading group was run by post-structuralists, postgraduate students of course, Joe Bristow, Geoff Gray and Judith Squires in the arts faculty.

Translations and discussions of Lacan's work were also appearing in literary and film journals: *Screen* and *Screen Education* were key secondary sources. The English department also housed feminist theorists such as Maud Ellmann, who was finishing her PhD, and they argued that the shift from biology to language effectively turned Lacanian psychoanalysis into a feminist-friendly account of how patriarchal oppression became embedded in the unconscious lifeworld of those subject to it. This meant that there was a convenient distance from the medical framing of his work; if Lacan was hostile to humanism, it was not because he was aiming to make psychoanalysis scientific. In fact, his critique of humanism was bound up with his critique of the IPA tradition, which I assumed at the time meant the tradition of psychoanalysis as clinical treatment.

It certainly looked like Lacan was ticking all the right boxes, attracting Marxists and feminists, and speaking about discourse as part of the symbolically-structured conditions in which we found ourselves. First stop in the *Écrits* reading group was his early paper on the mirror-stage, the narcissistic stage where we are confronted with images of loved- and hated-ones that we construct as counterparts to what we are beginning to imagine we are. Those counterparts are 'imagos' of the other that became patched together into what we henceforth take to be the core of our self. This looks like a developmental stage, but is really a launching pad into the Symbolic realm, a theatrical stage riddled with master-slave relations to fantasy-world others that stay with us through the rest of our lives.

Freud wrote about the 'narcissism of minor differences' in a wry comment on the way that people and groups differentiate themselves from rivals. These are differences that can quickly mutate from endearing likeness to aggressive self-assertion. In the reading group, we tussled over whether what Lacan would be talking about in his spin on Freud was 'aggression' as ahistorical universal instinct or 'aggressivity', the term he used to describe the phenomenological sense of threat from the other, which would depend on symbolic context. I wanted to avoid universalising claims about psychoanalytic subjectivity that would take us back to a psychological definition of development and social behaviour; historically-specific claims would be more in tune with possibilities for political change.

Maybe Freud, when commenting on the narcissism of minor differences, had in mind the kinds of conflicts revolving around apparently trivial doctrinal distinctions that had broken out in the IPA and its different component organisations. Those conflicts, ranging from the expulsion of Reich to the excommunication of Lacan, were certainly the site of exaggerated claims, with often disastrous consequences for psychoanalysis. Lacan's accusations against the IPA, characterising it as a bureaucratic apparatus that had sold out psychoanalysis when émigré analysts replanted it in Chicago and London after fleeing from the Nazis, were surely significant in the moves against him in 1953.

While the immediate stakes of that dispute were around the refusal of the IPA to recognise the new French psychoanalytic society Lacan founded – he had unwittingly excluded himself and colleagues by stepping out of the existing franchise organisation – there was already a bitter background to the dispute and the ten-year IPA 'investigation' into the affair, an investigation that lasted from 1953 to 1963. The break with the existing franchise organisation came after Lacan, who was nominally in charge of training, rejected a psychiatric syllabus proposed by loyal IPA colleagues.

That break with psychiatry, and with what Lacan saw as a psychological conception of the human subject, was bound up with the quasi-Hegelian reading of Freud he was already arguing for in the French society, and that was to be given more coherent shape by a linguistically-based return to Freud. For Lacan, bureaucratisation and psychologisation went hand-in-hand in the IPA, and he argued that this double-process, a double-problem, was tantamount to a betrayal of psychoanalysis. Just as psychoanalysts settling in the United States, anxious about their status in the New World, agreed to adapt psychoanalysis to the medical and individualising requirements of registration bodies there, so they turned psychoanalysis from being a practice of rebellious self-enquiry into an instrument of adaptation, something that proponents vaunted and Lacan sarcastically scorned as 'ego psychology'.

These were unavoidable political matters entangled with the psychoanalytic politics of the IPA as an institution; instead of equipping people to speak out, something that I saw as resonating with what Fromm and Reich were trying to do, psychoanalysis was now committing itself to turning out good, well-behaved citizens. Psychoanalysts before Lacan, including some of those keeping quiet about their radical politics after they relocated to the US, had made this kind of argument. Compatriots of Reich said as much, and Reich suffered before he died when he tried to stay true, in his own weird way, to a radical critique of the ego as the assumed rational centre of the individual. It involved what some historians such as Russell Jacoby, not a Lacanian, have referred to as 'the repression of psychoanalysis'.

Imaginary

There was a peculiar regression in the process of implanting psychoanalysis in the English-speaking world, from 'the line of the Symbolic' to 'the line of the Imaginary'. These cryptic formulations I picked up from the first psychoanalytic conference I went to, in June 1984, in Oxford. We will get to Cambridge and Jacques-Alain Miller in due course. This conference was called 'Approaching Lacan', organised by the Oxford Psycho-Analytical Forum, and compèred by Brett Kahr. There were around a hundred people there. The day was full of mysterious sayings, a surrealist short film by Manuel DeLanda called 'Raw Nerves: The Libidinal Economy of Filmus lnteruptus', and a performance by a student dressed up as Lacan, who strode around the front of the room wielding a cigar and speaking about psychosis. It was quite ridiculous.

John Forrester gave a clear measured introduction to Lacan, elaborating themes from his ground-breaking historical study *Language and the Origins of Psychoanalysis*, published four years before, in which it was clear that it was the 'turn to language' that was key to Freud's invention of his talking cure. Terry Eagleton lectured as a Marxist, complaining that while Lacan spoke of the human 'subject' he risked dissolving it in language: what we needed was some theory and practice of a 'collective subject' in order to change the world. I liked this. Toril Moi strode into the hall in motorcycle gear and released tresses of golden hair from her crash helmet, before launching into an argument that Lacan opened up new perspectives on femininity that celebrated surreal literary resistance to patriarchy. I liked that too. I had been at a talk in London the evening before on deconstruction by David Wood, then Jacques Derrida's most articulate voice in Britain. I told David about the Lacan conference, and so he turned up too, in order to tax the Lacanians again about their 'Phallogocentrism', the claim that Lacan not only privileged language as such, the logocentrism aspect, but a particular signifier in the Symbolic universe, the phallus.

The phallus is a privileged signifier for Lacanians, not the penis, and the distinction between the two is not even appreciated by all psychoanalysts. There is a story that Anna Freud once asked her father what the phallus was, and so he called her into his office, turned around, and took down his trousers. When he faced his daughter again to show her, Anna said "Oh, it's like a penis, only smaller." Fake news, just like the phallus is, and the pretend power that the phallus enjoys in our patriarchal Symbolic order, should be intimately linked to the motif of failure. Erica Burman, a feminist developmental psychologist, was at the deconstruction talk, and also came along to the Oxford conference to see this first Lacanian circus in Britain, and so there was a small radical contingent there during the day.

Richard Klein, a hard-core Lacanian, American – so there really were such beings – bewildered the audience, bewitched us with a little diagram scrawled on the blackboard. This diagram was Schema L, apparently pronounced, if you were a real Lacanian, as 'skaymah elle'. Read the next paragraphs in this chapter slowly.

Two diagonal lines criss-crossed the board. One line ran from a big 'S' top-left down to a big 'A' bottom-right. This was the line of the Symbolic. The other line ran from a little 'a' bottom-left up across to another little 'a' top-right. No, not exactly, this other 'a' top-right was marked with a little apostrophe mark, a prime, it was 'a-prime', a', this line was the line of the Imaginary. Get the picture? I didn't. This diagram was from early Lacan for whom the Imaginary was a lure, a lure of the image and an illusion of transparent understanding, a residue of the mirror-stage. There were a number of neat things about this diagram, maybe too many, too many for me. I don't know what everyone else made of it, but a little group of us shared notes afterwards, mystified by the way Richard Klein responded to almost every question by dramatically running his hand down from the bottom-left to top-right of the board, from 'a' to 'a-prime', declaring, in an emphatic clipped drawl, "that is the line of the Imaginary", sometimes saying nothing more than that.

Complications were layered upon complications. Hidden inside this diagram was the core of psychoanalysis. There at the top-right was 'S' for subject, the human subject, which was also marked in brackets '*Es*', the German original for 'It', which was translated into English as the 'id'. So, it would seem that what was most authentically human was something of the id, so far so Reichian, but then this 'S' subject was linked by the first diagonal line, the line of the Symbolic, to the big 'A', which I discovered was 'A' for '*Autre*', French for Other. This line had a direction arrow on it, coming from the Other, which was first a solid line marked 'unconscious' before it turned into dotted lines before arriving at the Subject. Perhaps this was indicating that the unconscious is the discourse of the Other. So, what was unconscious to us was bound up with the Symbolic, and Richard Klein clearly thought this line was a good line, one that we should have been talking about but that no one seemed to be getting to.

The second line cut across the first, and the little 'a' down in the bottom-left of the blackboard also précised that 'a' as the 'I' or ego (which in the French original is '*moi*') formed in an Imaginary relationship with a specular image of itself, the image of itself taking shape based on the image of the other, and there it is 'other' with a little a' up in the top-right. That is what the 'a-prime', a', stands for, '*autre*' with a little 'a' the little other. If the letter 'a' on three corners of the Schema L were each marked as 'o' for other, this might better capture something of the way that 'a-prime' also functions as object, enigmatic love object that the Subject searches for throughout its life, an enigmatic love object that was so important to the Subject during the formation of the ego during the mirror-stage. The Irish psychoanalyst Cormac Gallagher translates this *autre* as other on his useful 'lacaninireland' website. Most Lacanians retain 'a' and 'A' as the markers of otherness, however, in line with Lacan's and Miller's argument that this better facilitates the transmission of psychoanalysis as a constellation of 'mathemes' across actually-existing languages. The line of the Imaginary cuts down across the line of the Symbolic, blocking it, and so, we gathered from Richard Klein's contemptuous dismissal of our questions that repeatedly referred us to this line, was a bad thing, to be avoided.

What was sure was that psychoanalysis as a talking cure was supposed to be facilitating a kind of speech that would connect the Subject to the big Other along the line of the Symbolic. What was not so sure was whether that was equivalent to the release of the id energies in orgasmic delight, breaking through the repression that Reich and Reichians, interested in tackling 'character armour' and engaging in 'body work', would be aiming it. It was not. Or perhaps it could even then be seen as close enough to what Fromm was urging when he searched for a kind of relatedness between self and others, between self and society. It was not. I was very keen to read Lacan within frames of reference I already had, though, and the risk was that I would be simplifying and reducing Lacan to those conceptual grids.

It was easy to be transfixed by the Schema L. That is one reason I have not reproduced it as a figure in this book. You can look it up. It is too easy to be locked into a bewitched gaze on the figure, losing sight of the forms of language it traces. That, paradoxically, was precisely one of the dangers that Schema L was designed to draw attention to. It is itself an image, apparently direct and transparently open, summarising an array of different narrative accounts about the nature of the human subject. As an image it repeats the experience the infant has of being confronted with a specular image of itself in the mirror-stage, an image it finds in an actual mirror or in the mirroring responses of an adult caregiver, using that image to form itself as an ego and then to defend itself against a host of hallucinatory surreal images of the fragmented body pulled in different directions by the drives. This Schema L is in the realm of the Imaginary, a diagram that makes sense to us in the line of the Imaginary. And it renders an aspect of psychoanalytic theory understandable to us, as if we could break through what Lacan calls 'the wall of language', even as if Richard Klein could convey to us exactly what Lacan wanted to say and as if he could communicate with us as he tried to explain what Lacanian psychoanalysis is.

It fails, of course, and perhaps that itself is another aspect of the diagram that fascinates us, well, fascinates Lacanians and wannabe Lacanians. It fails because we still need it to be elaborated within language for it to make sense to us. It is of the Imaginary, but also of the Symbolic, framed by the Symbolic, just as the infant is when looking in a mirror or into their caregiver's face, or sensing the responses of a first other through other modalities of sense. You need the Symbolic alongside the Imaginary, and you cannot do without elements of Imaginary understanding in order to maintain some level of connection – 'recognition' Hegelians and Lacanians would say – between speakers and listeners, or between writers and readers. Here in Oxford, we could withstand the mysterious presentation and cryptic answers of Richard Klein, Lacanian, because the event was symbolically framed, ordered within the symbolic frame of a particular stretch of time – we knew it would soon be over and that we would have space to step aside from it and puzzle about it with our friends – and the frame of the day's conference was, after all, that it was about Lacan.

We knew what we were letting ourselves in for when we signed up for this first Lacanian conference in Britain, knew that we would be treated to a display of rebellious complaint directed at the symbolic domination of psychoanalysis in Britain by the British Psychoanalytical Society, avatar of the IPA. We knew this intervention was a Lacanian manoeuvre. This is very unlike what an infant knows when it looks in the mirror to enter the Imaginary, and then starts to speak, enters the Symbolic. We already, unlike the infant, had some compass points, something you need to defend yourself against the unexpected, the uncanny and against the third register, which Lacan called the Real. It is sometimes said that Lacan's work can be divided into three phases, focusing first on the Imaginary, then on the Symbolic, and then on the Real. The 'later Lacan' of the Real was brought to fruition in late Lacan. He died in 1981, and it was then that Jacques-Alain Miller took the reins of his school.

Real

We were here to see Miller speak in Cambridge in January 1985. Now we are here. This two-day conference on 'Transmission and Psychoanalysis' was organised by the Cambridge Psychoanalytic Study Group. It was a much smaller event, about half the number that had been in Oxford, but this was the real deal, bringing together Lacanians to hear the leader of the pack, Jacques-Alain Miller. There were a few detractors, like Malcolm Pines, and some outsiders, like my friend Geoff Gray, a Southampton philosophy PhD student from the *Écrits* reading group, and me. A bedraggled French philosopher Daniel Sibony stood unhappily at the side of the room, shunned by the Lacanians because, it was whispered to us, Miller objected to his presence as he was not a psychoanalyst. Pines sat defiant as tribune of the IPA on a table at the back. We trekked through the snow for the second day of the conference and huddled together in Trinity College in the room where the philosopher of language, Ludwig Wittgenstein, had reputedly threatened the positivist Karl Popper with a poker. Before he became a philosopher, Popper worked in progressive psychoanalytic welfare organisations run by followers of the ex-psychoanalyst Alfred Adler, but he turned against all forms of psychoanalysis because they were unscientific, and turned against Marxism for much the same reason.

This room in Trinity was a good setting to talk about recent psychoanalysis as part of a turn to language. Miller, standing by the side of an immense fireplace, spent some time waxing lyrical during his concluding talk for the conference on 'The Mainstream of Lacan's Thought', about the College as the site of the famous poker contest, and about the Trinity. Aha, I thought; the Symbolic, Imaginary and Real. He then launched into a clearly structured account of three key elements of Lacan's work.

The first element was, of course, Freud, and Lacan's famous 'return to Freud', which excavated an authentic psychoanalytic concern with the unconscious, the unconscious as structured like a language. It was easy enough to babble on about language in literary theory, but the return to Freud also meant taking seriously infantile sexuality and trauma that erupted from time to time as indications that there was something real at stake in psychoanalysis. To speak of 'the Real' as a third register in Lacanian theory was not to pretend that we could plumb its depths with the right instruments but to attend to its effects, to the way it disrupted Symbolic forms and Imaginary communication.

There was a clear bid here by Miller to locate Lacan in the mainstream of psychoanalytic thought, to pit Lacan against and alongside the IPA. This conference was a precursor to the development of Lacanian psychoanalysis in Britain, and intended as a direct challenge to the attempts by the IPA to pretend that there was no such thing in the English-speaking world, attempts to perpetuate the exclusion of Lacanian work that had begun in 1953. Pines rose to the bait with his faux-psychoanalytic interpretations of Lacan, Miller and his followers wanted to be persecuted. We were at the heart of contemporary psychoanalytic politics.

Miller then turned to structuralism, a second element that was important to the turn back to language as a central defining feature of Freud's work, but one that should not be overestimated, should be contextualised. Structuralism and so-called 'post-structuralism' had been overarching theoretical frames in our *Écrits* reading group, and it was the central organising principle in University of London extramural studies classes I had been attending to a get a grip on what Lacan, Foucault and Derrida were up to. Our arguments about how to read the mirror-stage paper in the *Écrits* revolved around the hard-line structuralist argument that was to be found in the structural anthropology of Claude Lévi-Strauss, that there were universal structures of kinship in which women were treated as objects of exchange. If that was the case, then it was hard to see where feminism came in, other than as continuing the critique of Freud that had been articulated so well by writers like Kate Millett.

Perhaps what came after structuralism, such as internal critiques by writers like Derrida and Foucault, would shift us on from the rather reactionary anthropological arguments made by Lévi-Strauss. Miller sidestepped this in his talk, focusing instead on the structural linguistics of Ferdinand de Saussure as something that gave us the conceptual tools to read Freud as a theorist of language. Saussure differentiated between the signifier or sound-image and the signified or concept, two components of signs that comprise the Symbolic order. We had interpreted this in Southampton as meaning that signifiers were the anchor points of consciousness, what Freud called 'word presentations', while signifieds were mental concepts, the 'thing presentations' that could be subject to repression, in the unconscious. This was not exactly right, but it worked well enough as a ladder up into Lacan's work that we could then kick away later.

The signifier and signified were, Saussure argued, as two sides of a sheet of paper, intimately connected to each other, but – and this was something the 'post-structuralists' made hay of – there was a perpetual sliding of signifieds under signifiers. That slippage was what the linguist Roman Jakobson described in his account of metaphor and metonymy, which Lacan reinterpreted as a linguistic account of repression and desire. To say that Freud was the 'father' of psychoanalysis, for example, is to use a metaphor that replaces an account of the transmission of clinical research with an image of a patriarchal family lineage. You might then believe you need fathers in psychoanalytic theory, and fall in line with the idea that the issue of generational succession in the psychoanalytic movement is naturally from father to son, or, when there was no son, son-in-law. Metaphor replaces one term for another, pushing it out of the way, even out of consciousness. Metonymy, on the other hand, displaces attention from one term to another, just as desire drives us from one object to another in a fruitless search for satisfaction. We read Freud, don't quite get it, and then Lacan, and it doesn't make sense, and chase from one theorist to another hoping that they will come up with the goods, carried along in a metonymical movement across the chain of signifiers.

Here also was one of the manifestations of the ineluctable fruitlessness and emptiness of desire that Lacanians dubbed 'lack'. This structuralist account of the nature of the Symbolic was also, among other things, a battering ram against the ego psychologists of the IPA who were still busy promising their patients that they could be made whole and healthy and happy. Miller was settling political scores while putting Lacan on the map in British psychoanalysis. My mind was whizzing, and I was patching-in ideas I had already read about in Lacanian theory to make sense of what Miller was saying, patching them in to fill the gaps in the argument, gaps for me, gaps, as tears in the fabric of the argument where I was losing the thread.

The third element of Lacan's work was one I associated with the Imaginary, what Miller called 'the subject'. You should take care here with my attempt to make sense of what I heard. I contrasted this account with the ways that psychologists in my own university department spoke about 'the subject' in their experiments to describe the participants they treated as objects. This philosophical conception of the subject Miller spoke of was not reduced to the psychological push-pull mechanism of the mind nor to the 'conflict-free sphere of the ego' in contemporary 'ego psychology'. It encompassed what there was of us as human beings in the unconscious, repressed reminders of desire. I associated it with the Imaginary because we seemed here to be in the realm of the master-slave dialectic, a quasi-anthropological notion Alexandre Kojève retrieved from Hegel's work in the Paris lectures that Lacan and existentialist writers like Sartre attended.

But it was much more than that. It exceeds such expectations, attempts to fix the problems posed by the image of master and slave. This is also the realm of the unconscious, not deliberate combat, of what lies beyond who we think we are. We are subjects. If you take seriously Lacan's image of the Subject as presented in the Schema L, then the S at the top left-hand corner of the diagram is itself divided. It is split there, where we imagine that it is whole, just as it is split and distributed across the four corners of the Schema L. The Subject is not of the Imaginary but blocked, betrayed by it.

I relaxed, too comfortable I suspect, as I heard Miller talk about this subject as something close to the subject of the existentialist tradition. In Hegel's master-slave dialectic the question is who is to be master, a subject, and who is to give recognition to that master and thus be positioned as object. The master falls to the position of slave when he realises that he is dependent on the slave, that he craves recognition. Here in Trinity College the battle was not with pokers but with language, a battle for recognition, and a political battle over who would be recognised as psychoanalyst.

There was something uncannily familiar about all this from my time in Trotskyist sect squabbles, and all the more so because the organisational battles were also played out on a global scale. There are many warring psychoanalytic organisations, it is not only a Lacanian problem, but I had heard more than once that the similarity between Lacanians and Trotskyists is that it takes only one person to found an organisation, that when there are two they declare an 'international', and that when there are three there is a split. The political is personal in this process as institutional rivalries intersect with individual strategies to cling on to power.

The bureaucratic manoeuvres by the IPA, intended to exclude Lacan and the formation of a new international organisation later headed by his son-in-law Jacques-Alain Miller to promote Lacanian psychoanalysis, were bound up with petty personal intrigues. It could not be otherwise, for this was a battle for Freud using structuralism as a weapon on the terrain of the subject. I was attracted to this but appalled by it, still sure that I should avoid psychoanalysis and, more so, psychoanalytic politics. It was another lesson about problems with Freud and the institutions he founded, giving me another good reason to keep well out of it. Many people steer clear of psychoanalysis because it refers to things they do not like to think about, and also because of the interminable internal squabbling that marks its institutions, but then something about it is fascinating, attractive as it is appalling, and that, the stuff of unconscious, is what pulls us back to it again, and incites us to want to tell others about it.

4

TEACHING

Avoiding analytic practice

A fourth strong warning against psychoanalysis comes in the form it takes when it is taught, and we should beware of the way that educational institutions reinforce rationalist models of the mind that look like psychoanalysis, but systematically distort what Freud and his followers were trying to describe. I will show you why I still avoided psychoanalytic clinical practice, after having discovered how efficiently it can be neutralised and absorbed into psychotherapeutic attempts to adapt people to society, adaptation of individuals that the university insidiously demands of us. Here is another reason I kept away from psychoanalysis for so long.

Feeling

Freud muses in one of his papers about what he would include in the curriculum in any future 'College of Psychoanalysis'. Although he does include some topics related to his own neurophysiological and psychiatric career, pride of place is given to the arts, to literature and mythology. It is this kind of reflection on teaching that sometimes leads Freudians to argue that psychoanalysis should not be viewed as a natural science at all, but as one of the human sciences. This was the line taken by Bruno Bettelheim shortly before he died, when he was urging analysts to return to the meaning of Freud and to a more faithful translation into English from the original German that would do justice to the humanistic aspect of his work. The discipline of psychology did not figure among the subjects Freud included in his wish list. But some versions of psychoanalysis were included in the psychology undergraduate degree at Manchester Polytechnic when I arrived there for my first teaching post in 1985.

The third-year option 'Counselling' was on my timetable, as were theories of personality on a counselling diploma course, and I would have some input on a master's course in art education. There were many other fragments of courses I taught in my first years in Manchester when anything approaching psychoanalysis was out of the question. I had hoped to bring in some ideas from a radical psychology book called *Changing the Subject*, which was published in 1984 and which a very small group of postgraduates, on the edge of the discipline, rallied around as virtually the only voice for something completely different. Most of the five co-authors had been active in the journal *Ideology and Consciousness*. The book by Julian Henriques, Wendy Hollway, Cathy Urwin, Couze Venn and Valerie Walkerdine blended arguments from Jacques Derrida and deconstruction, from Michel Foucault, whose influence was signalled in the subtitle 'Psychology, Social Regulation and Subjectivity', and from Jacques Lacan. Lacan underpinned the main psychoanalytic argument of the book combined with ideas from the 'British tradition' IPA analyst, Melanie Klein.

The art education master's course, which ran from six to nine at night, and where the students were stressed, exhausted schoolteachers, was the only place where I could talk about Freud. I entertained them with analyses of Greek and Roman statuary, which claimed that the absence of body parts was part of the attraction – Melanie Klein funnelled through art historian Peter Fuller on the infant's relation to bits of the body was useful here – and with Freud's own interpretation of Leonardo da Vinci's memories of childhood and of the hidden image of a vulture in the painting 'The Virgin and Child with St Anne'. The art teachers groaned and objected, but at least they were willing to play along and speculate about what other interpretations might work better.

The counselling diploma course leader, the (appropriately-named) Frank, Frank Ashton, wanted standard psychological personality theories, such as behaviourist social learning theory and biological accounts of differential reactive activity in the brain's limbic system, taught to his students. No Freud, that was not psychology. But even the psychological theories were fairly useless in the context of the diploma, which was avowedly humanistic. I guess my contribution was designed to set up those mechanistic theories so they could be easily knocked down again later. The focus on thinking could then be replaced with a focus on feeling. This psychotherapeutic framework pitted itself against psychology but also effectively complemented its rival discipline. I was to learn that it was also antithetical to psychoanalysis.

I managed to avoid teaching the behaviourist third of the counselling option on the psychology degree, risking the job at interview when I said I had an ethical objection to it, and so was landed with the humanistic third. The psychoanalytic third, which was mainly Kleinian, was already taken; the tutor, a jolly, racist, sexist old guy, who told me that he thought about how happy he was to be a psychologist every morning he got out of bed, had run it for years and would hang on to it until he retired. Not long to go I thought, I hoped.

Meantime, I could distance myself from the positivist theories I taught in the straight laboratory-experimental psychology courses, teach those theories as stories, discourses, and hint at the Foucauldian critique of laboratory-experimentation, categorisation and surveillance that *Changing the Subject* described. Here, in mainstream psychology, was one obvious side of the reduction to the individual that the book decried as 'the rational unitary subject'. The humanistic image of the subject, in which there was also a critique of rationalist models of the mind, was going to be a harder nut to crack, especially in a counselling option that was supposed to link with practice.

Some psychology students did, quite understandably, turn to some kind of phenomenological approach, an approach that began with experience and valued it instead of dismissing it as much psychological quantitative research tended to do. Phenomenology promised to go 'back to the things themselves' – that was Edmund Husserl's formulation – and so it did seem to reach back to what psychology left out. Husserl died in 1938, a year before Freud, and was a touchstone for phenomenological and then existentialist debates in Germany and France, debates that included figures ranging from Martin Heidegger, his student, to Kojève and Sartre.

I remembered that, back in Southampton, the feminist post-structuralist Maud Ellmann insisted, in line with Freud's own psychoanalytic argument, that it was a mistake to engage in a kind of phenomenological study that aimed to retrieve a true consciousness of the meaning of a dream. Instead, what was of interest to psychoanalysis was in what escaped any kind of 'psychological' description, and especially so in Lacan's 'return to Freud'. What we are confronted with in psychoanalysis is a process of repression, the *process* not the search for something under the surface that has been repressed. That poses a big problem for the forms of psychology that take any notice of what Freud said, and is the diametric opposite of psychological accounts of his work in the textbooks that portray the unconscious mind as if it were some kind of box with unpleasant memories and perceptions locked inside it.

By now I knew that David Stafford-Clark's *What Freud Really Said*, peddled in Newcastle and Plymouth as a quick easy primer of psychoanalysis, was riddled with errors – a psychiatric reframing of Freud that used the term 'subconscious' and that told us Freud had described the Electra Complex as a feminine alternative to the Oedipus Complex, when in fact Freud had actually explicitly distanced himself from this Jungian formulation. If Stafford-Clark was to be believed, psychoanalysts try to dig things out of the unconscious with their interpretations.

I had invited Maud Ellmann to speak about the dreamwork at a lunchtime seminar in the psychology department at Southampton. A small gaggle of supporters from literature and philosophy came along to her talk and the few psychologists who turned up reacted with polite, uncomprehending silence. This was not the Freud they knew. They were more comfortable with the idea that the unconscious and our dream lives are under the surface, and that if a psychologist were to ever take such things seriously it would be with the aim of delving into them, uncovering them and finding out what they 'really' meant. This was of a piece with the popular romanticising of childhood as the place where innocent dreams were produced before hard reality was drummed in. My boy Ben, when he was ten years old, voiced this perfectly one day when I was describing a conference talk I had heard about dreams; he asked, puzzled, "do adults dream too?". The *Changing the Subject* take on this, in line with Lacan's reading of Freud, was that the gap between conscious and unconscious was formed as we entered language, and that dreams appeared as an expression of that gap; and so psychoanalysis provided one of the ways of describing the nature of the human being as a kind of irrational, divided subject, always so, not amenable to being tidied up.

Surely, the humanists in Manchester, my new home, told me, the subject yearned to heal itself. There was a little joke around at the time, part of a series, which asked how many therapists it takes to change a light bulb, and answered that it only took one but the light bulb must really want to change. When Frank vetted me for the counselling diploma teaching, he emphasised that this desire to change was intimately linked to the knowledge the subject already had about what was wrong and what they needed to do. You could see this in counselling practice, he said. Well, I didn't know a thing about the practice, so I kept to the theory, and framed it in terms I already knew, unwittingly keeping in line with an academic psychological approach to teaching about such things.

The unavoidable first stop was Carl Rogers, mainstay of a humanistic 'person-centred' approach. This approach was so person-centred that it refused to refer to patients or clients: 'persons' were at the centre of the theory, and at the centre of the person was the 'self'. Even this 'organismic self' was treated like a little person by Rogers who was trained and taught as a clinical psychologist. Genuineness, warmth and empathy would nurture this self in therapy, releasing it from the defensive patterns that both protected it and imprisoned it, patterns of response that were learned during a childhood in which such love and recognition had been withheld.

Rogers repeated elements of the master-slave dialectic described by Hegel, but as a potentially much smoother individual developmental process that could and should have a much happier outcome. At the heart of the master-slave dialectic, remember, was a battle for recognition, and there was no guarantee that this battle would ever end. While Hegel and Kojève looked to some kind of resolution at the end of history, Rogers was content with arriving at mutual recognition, a win-win situation in which two fully-formed subjects would emerge. Someone who had been given recognition by a significant other, if not very early on by a parent figure then by a therapist later in life, could, Rogers argued, become 'actualised' as what he called a 'fully-functioning person'.

The counsellor should themselves, of course, be a fully-functioning person for this to work out well in therapy, and at least be well on the road to having actualised themselves. It was difficult to know how to convey how important this was without falling back on moralistic injunctions to be a good person, open to experience, and open to others. Rogers himself first trained as a Christian minister, and the quasi-Hegelian story of each soul finding itself in relation to others was there with him all his life, even if he did later become an atheist and give up on what Hegel called the 'world spirit'.

For Rogers and for the tradition of humanistic person-centred approaches to counselling and psychotherapy that developed after him, the touchstone was feeling, something that could be gestured at as something intrinsically good in teaching but that could never be made completely evident to students. Feelings as lying in the domain of the organismic self were beyond the empirical evidence base of psychological theory, of course, and while I was sceptical about psychology I was not a humanist. This meant that when I talked about feelings, and how Rogers valued them so much, I too was on the side of the sceptics. I was part of the problem, a radical humanist might say, rather than part of the solution; but an overarching aspect of this problem was the academic disciplinary frame in which I was trying to speak and maintain some distance from humanism.

Our lectures were interleaved with visiting speakers from counselling services, something that made the option very popular with students because it did connect what we were describing with practice, and most of these services used versions of Rogerian person-centred theory in their training. Volunteers from the Marriage Guidance Council, renamed 'Relate' to sidestep the accusation that they were dead set on patching up families, were regular guests on the course, as were Cruse, a bereavement service, and Rape Crisis. These volunteers were all decent, conscientious people willing to give of their time to make a pitch for their service and raise consciousness about their work. I could well imagine speaking to these lovely people about my problems and agreeing that I really should take responsibility for my feelings, acknowledge them, and work with them rather than against them.

This approach to communication and consensus made sense in the context of Relate because a couple deciding whether to heal differences or separate from each other needed not only to express what they felt but also learn to listen to the other person. However, as the years went on, I noticed that the speakers were referring more and more to family dynamics, systems of relationships that couples were tangled up in, and to unconscious patterns. It was true that Rogers himself was profoundly influenced by pop-psychoanalysis – quasi-unconscious needs were masked by defence mechanisms and suchlike, blocks to self-actualisation – and these references to the unconscious were classically Freudian. Speakers described, sometimes only over coffee outside the teaching session, how their 'Continuing Professional Development' programmes were leading them in that direction. It seemed as if Rogers was the phenomenological first stop and basic platform for therapy in the service while psychoanalysis was seen as more advanced.

Similarly, in the case of Cruse, bereavement called for active listening so that the sense of loss could be 'worked through', but fairly soon it became clear that this working through was also framed within psychoanalytic theory as a work of mourning, mourning the lost love object. The first person-centred requirement for sensitive work with the bereaved was increasingly being elaborated during the late 1980s by Freudian theory, as volunteers underwent more advanced training. An exception to this process of uptake of quasi-psychoanalytic discourse was Rape Crisis. There was understandable anger among volunteers in that service at the stereotyping of feminine experience in psychoanalysis, particularly the claim that women's masochistic position in relation to sex might mean that at some unconscious level they desired the violence they were subjected to, that they were asking for it.

We knew there was just such a danger with psychoanalytic theory in domestic violence services where the return of women to violent partners was sometimes explained by way of masochistic attachment. The out-feminists from Rape Crisis instead were shifting their focus to endemic violence against women in society, a manifestation of male power, and eventually, in later years, spent much of their time in the visiting speaker sessions insisting, against protests from women students, that no woman was safe, and should never feel safe. Safety was an illusion. These sessions were the most disturbing ones in the counselling option, for they ran against the prevailing assumption that counsellors could learn about what people felt and help them feel better. Rape Crisis was, instead, part of a collective political project, and their interventions increasingly drew attention to the limits of psychoanalysis taught in an academic context, psychoanalysis that very quickly and easily turned into a reductively individualistic version of psychology. My attempts to teach psychoanalysis in that context again warned me off clinical practice.

Thinking

My first experience of a fully therapeutic frame in practice was in an assertiveness-training course in Manchester in which we were told by the facilitator "Your feelings are your friends". Not mine, I thought. The idea was that if you had bad feelings that held you back from asking for what you wanted, from asserting yourself, then these were false 'racket feelings', which played off from genuine self-friendly feelings that should guide you to the good things in life. It was when the facilitator started drawing diagrams on the board to picture the difference between healthy assertive relationships and manipulative ones in which racket feelings were in charge that I realised what theoretical framework was being deployed here. This time it wasn't Jacques Lacan's ideas on the board but those of Eric Berne.

Eric Berne's Transactional Analysis (TA) is used as a fully-fledged therapeutic approach in the clinic as well as an organisational tool to identify patterns of interaction between employees and their managers, used to ensure compliance in the US tax collection service, for example, or in air force and army bases, and in assertiveness training. The Manchester course facilitator, Suzy Lendrum, used the approach to keep order and explained to us, the punters, how we could use it to bring order to our lives and relationships. We were each asked to describe what phrases had power over us when used by others we wanted to be assertive to. I noticed that the phrase 'you know' said accusingly in arguments infuriated and paralysed me, that fury must be a racket feeling I guess, and Suzy dutifully wrote the phrase up on the board with the other phrases that the poor saps in the group had offered up during this first session. "So, Ian, you don't like it when someone says 'they know'," she said, and I thought that, yes, it did seem a bit daft when you put it like that.

There wasn't time, and it would have been out of place, to argue that, no, there was something about the way it was said in the context of a relationship, where it was being implied that I was being deliberately stupid, obtuse. I wasn't assertive enough to make the point. I wondered if this was the same or different from someone who had a problem, and couldn't find a way through it, being told that they really did know what the solution was, that if they followed their feelings or had a genuine, warm and empathic listener to actualise themselves, they would be able to voice what they already knew deep down. We practised in pairs and small groups asking for things and repeating phrases, 'broken record' this was called, to avoid being blocked or distracted. I imagined repeating such phrases: there were people I knew who would be enraged by this, and would make me pay. Drawing attention to their rage as a racket feeling would be out of the game.

It all seemed down to me, just as it seemed down to the person in a Rogerian approach to receive the recognition that was due to them and stop behaving like a slave to others. Power in relationships that reproduced power in the family – the kind of thing that Wilhelm Reich had drawn attention to – or that replicated power running through society, which Foucault tracked, wasn't taken seriously in either of these humanist approaches. For Rogers and for Berne it was up to the individual to stop being a victim and speak out about what they felt or knew to be right for them. When the course was over I described what had gone on in the evening at a restaurant to my partner's mother. She said, "Could you use your assertiveness skills to ask them to turn down the music so we can hear ourselves speak." I did.

During my first years of counselling option teaching, however, I latched on to Berne's approach. It was perfect for the humanist strand of the course; it was a more complex elaboration of Rogers' ideas, and it smuggled in psychoanalytic ideas. Berne was on course to become a psychoanalyst but, in 1956, after fifteen years of lectures and supervision, he gave up after being messed around, as he saw it, by the San Francisco Training Institute, which had refused him membership. Berne quickly cobbled together his own theory, which turned the Freudian categories of 'id', 'ego' and 'superego' into a more easily accessible common-sense account of the tangled 'transactions' that people make with each other from 'child', 'adult' or 'parent' ego states, which then hook one or more of those ego states in another person. The beauty of TA lies in the way that everyday interactions can be decoded. Berne provided detailed accounts of how people spoke to others or even laughed if they were in one ego state or another. The parent ego state laughs with a patronising 'ho ho', for example, while the adult gives a rational and reasonable 'ha ha', and the child ego state expresses its infantile character with 'hee hee'.

Berne popularised his theory through best-selling books like *Games People Play*, which described the different games or 'scripts' that enable people to get along with each other so they both get something out of the interaction, so they both, as Berne would say, get 'strokes'. These 'strokes' seemed to describe discrete units of recognition, recognition felt as warm appreciation from another human being who was treating you as if you were a subject rather than an as object in interaction. Memorable phrases to sum up human needs like 'folks need strokes' helped TA sell this banalised psychoanalytic theory to the general public, though it was an approach that was often looked down upon by psychologists, partly because it was much more popular than their own rather more boring and thoroughly-tested-to-death theories. I searched for empirical studies and critiques of TA in vain, and when I failed to find any, found that vaguely reassuring.

In some countries, Germany for instance, TA isn't viewed by the professional registration bodies as a therapy but as a form of education because the TA 'therapist' usually makes great use of marker boards and flip charts on which they sketch out the dysfunctional patterns of interaction that their clients should avoid, and spell out what would be more healthy. While there is recognition that we are divided into adult, parent and child, the aim is to integrate experience and so facilitate rational adult communication between undivided subjects.

While Rogers had a much-expanded notion of the 'self' that could, ideally, be actualised as an 'organismic' self and was rather critical of rationality, Berne prioritised the adult ego state as the site for rational evaluation. The claim that your feelings are your friends looked at first to be in tune with a Rogerian humanistic argument about the self, but, when it came down to it, once you could sort out racket feelings from real feelings then it was the ego that was in charge. The emphasis was on thinking rather than feeling, and would-be psychologists found that reassuring. And, best of all, it offered a fuller box of tricks than did the relatively limited 'core conditions' in Rogerian person-centred therapy.

I liked this theory a lot when I had to teach humanistic approaches, because at least TA seemed as much concerned with the 'transactions' as the things going on inside the mind of the client. It was clear and prescriptive – you knew what was what and you knew what you had to do to bring people back into line with each other – how their lines of communication might run adult to adult, and this is very much in the way that communication in the class was supposed to. The beauty of it was that it was a profoundly educational approach, suited for teaching counselling students if not directly useful for their practice when they graduated.

Maybe it was useful in practice. My experience of it in assertiveness training was fun, but I suspected that if those in power were wise to the rules, there was no reason why they should not anticipate techniques like the 'broken record' and know very well how to give or withhold the 'strokes' that they were told people crave. It seemed like it could be a route to empowerment in some contexts, but in others a recipe for dependence. It could well make psychoanalytic ideas more accessible for all, but it could also, by the same token, turn popularised psychoanalysis into a tool of control; and relaying it as a theory of the self through academic psychology gave it a seal of approval to make it more of a liability.

Balancing

We didn't have speakers from the local Transactional Analysis centre, but it was a popular choice as a 'service' that the students could evaluate as their class assignment for the option. The TA people seemed more willing to talk to students, perhaps because some of those students were already beginning to enrol in short courses at the centre, and it was easier to get access to than to hard-pressed voluntary services besieged by clients in distress. TA training organisations seemed even more for the 'worried well' than the person-centred support services.

Unfortunately there were no services offering a menu of approaches to be found in the *Innovative Therapy in Britain* book, edited by John Rowan and Windy Dryden, that I began using when teaching the counselling option. I wanted to try to break the deadlock between the three main components of the option and to open it out to new approaches, such as Gestalt therapy, feminist therapy or psychosynthesis, approaches that were each broadly humanistic, at least in the rendering of them selected by Rowan and Dryden. One common theme in that book, in which practitioners were tasked to describe a client experience of their own particular framework, was that the client felt better and then decided to train as a therapist themselves. This was unproblematic, of course, in a counselling option that took for granted the idea that more training for more people must be a good thing, but it alerted me to something that cynics might call 'pyramid selling' in therapeutic services. Why not, if you really believe it works, persuade other people to join in, spread the good news?

The student evaluation of a chosen service did, in the best of cases, enable a break from the quantitative laboratory-experimental studies that they were taught in most of the other parts of the degree course, but the qualitative aspect of the evaluation – some kind of ethnographic description and an interview with staff – also led them into a tangle of contradictions. Were they to believe what people in the service said if it struck the student-investigator as being intuitively right, or should they subject what they were told to some kind of rigorous empirical investigation? This difficult choice went alongside an equally difficult decision as to whether they should take the theoretical framework that was being employed on good coin, or whether they should draw on what they knew of the variety of different frameworks taught across the option.

In practice, the students rarely plumped for a framework that was different from the one being described to them. Sometimes they took the risky path of uncritically relaying what they had been told in the interviews with workers or volunteers, merely suggesting that there be better access to the service and, of course, more funding. That was a risky path because they might then be penalised for failing to stand back and *really* 'evaluate' the claims. Often they resorted to the safest path, which was to conclude that a combination of the different perspectives they had heard about might provide a more balanced therapeutic approach. A similar response was demanded of them in the end-of-year examinations. The only way they could demonstrate that they were thinking critically about a particular theoretical framework they were describing – whether that was humanistic, psychoanalytic or cognitive/behavioural – would be to bring in elements of rival frameworks. The 'compare and contrast' questions on the exam paper provided the most explicit platform for this response.

There were, of course, ready-to-hand rhetorical devices in psychotherapeutic discourse to warrant this balanced approach, a balanced approach that acknowledged the feeling and thinking elements of a problem, as well as the experiential, cognitive and behavioural elements of a solution. 'Eclectic' was one possibility, except it implied that different competing approaches might be simply cobbled together, and so the most popular term became 'integrative'. Notice that the 'integration' of different models also presupposes an integration of the different aspects of the human subject that are differentially weighted in different models. To say that you are 'integrative' answers to the demand for a balance between different competing frameworks, and to some kind of balancing between external and internal forces as well as between different kinds of internal force.

This is ego psychology in action with a vengeance, ego psychology in an academic context that expects that the taking of sides indicates that you are unbalanced; when it comes down to it, that you are un-therapeutic. The attempt to connect with practice thus failed because we were asking our students to keep a distance from what they described. What psychoanalytic ideas there were in the different approaches we included in the option were drawn into the academic frame and transformed by that frame into something else. Then it seemed safer to avoid it altogether.

Not only should we avoid psychoanalytic practice because it is unscientific, sexist and mired in political-institutional infighting, but also because, whenever you tried to teach it to others, you inevitably turned it into something worse. What, you might ask, was there to like in all this. The next four chapters try to answer that question, describing how I turned from avoiding psychoanalysis to engaging with it.

5

SOCIETY

Engaging with the British tradition

Psychoanalytic ideas provide quite convincing explanations for the intersection between social processes and personal responses to those processes. That was enough of a hook. I was being drawn in. This chapter shows how the link between psychoanalysis and sociology in the British tradition was worked at by those on the left keen to understand the relationship between personal threat and institutional defences. I focus on one attempt to draw on clinical experience to understand politics, a project that viewed 'free association' as the free development of each as a condition for the free development of all.

Before

"My wife," he said. These were the first two words Mike Rustin uttered as he opened the first 'Psychoanalysis and the Public Sphere' conference at North East London Polytechnic, NELP, in Stratford. It would be mean to blame Rustin for such implicit and assumed heteronormative framing of the conference – the male speaker marks his partner as wife – and we need a broader conception of the unconscious to be able to treat such statements as 'symptomatic'. These are the social arrangements that make psychoanalysis possible and thus attractive to those who would want to use the framework to cure others or interpret social phenomena. It was an innocent beginning, which assumed significance after the event, in the light of other discussions during the two days at NELP. I felt a twinge of guilt. I had applied for a lectureship there in psychology the year before, got the job, prevaricated, and then turned it down to stay in Manchester. This conference was hosted by a sociologist, Rustin, and a Darwin scholar, Bob Young. It promised to give a different disciplinary and political angle on psychoanalysis and a reason to find out what was going on.

I had travelled to London the night before, and had hardly slept as the howling winds of the Great Storm of 1987 wailed through the north of the city. Rustin, an academic sociologist at NELP, who also had a position at the Tavistock Clinic – a Mecca for the IPA tradition in psychoanalysis – had hardly made it out to Stratford either. He was telling us what his wife, Margaret Rustin, a psychoanalytic psychotherapist at the Tavistock, had said to him about the weather. We will return to Mike and Bob and the gang in due course, but first we follow some threads that led me there that October, the beginning of my third year of teaching, when I had found a way of engaging with psychoanalysis.

Some of the undergraduate students doing qualitative research projects began to show an interest in psychoanalysis and this encouraged me to think about running a final year option on 'Psychoanalysis and Society'. In that option we covered three main currents of work in psychoanalysis: first the so-called 'British tradition' of psychoanalysis, which included the work of Melanie Klein, Donald Winnicott and Wilfred Bion; then the German tradition of work in the Frankfurt School, which ranged from Wilhelm Reich to Jürgen Habermas; finishing with French contributions in and around Jacques Lacan. I taught the theories, but I also wanted to explore how these theories functioned within the different cultural-historical traditions that gave rise to them, and, though we had less time to do this, to reflect on how they had some status themselves as competing discourses that described subjectivity. I began writing the lectures before the option ran, thinking of them as chapters in a book – that did eventually appear, ten years later, as *Psychoanalytic Culture: Psychoanalytic Discourse in Western Society*.

The French and German frames for psychoanalytic theory were now pretty familiar to me from the reading groups and extramural studies courses I had taken while doing my PhD in Southampton, but the work of Melanie Klein and co. was a more daunting field, partly because Mrs Klein, an émigré to Britain from Germany before the Second World War, herself was such a forbidding figure and partly because those who spoke about her seemed a little too dead certain that she was right. The German writers in the Frankfurt School embedded psychoanalysis in a reflexive critique of the nature of the Western Enlightenment in which an emphasis on the ego was treated as part of the problem; and the French Lacanians were already talking about psychic processes as structured within discourse. But Klein was really talking about things going on inside the mind of the infant, before, beyond and beneath language; it was the worst of psychoanalytic discourse, closed, hermetic, with little quarter given to those who tried to contest it.

It was all the more surprising, perhaps, that Klein had become the focus of sociologists and then radicals in sociology and psychotherapy training, who saw in her work something social and progressive. In comparison with the Winnicott-focused 'object relations' strand of work in British psychoanalysis, with which it is often confused, Klein's approach was actually profoundly asocial. For her, it was not actual object relations or first encounters with the maternal object as object of love that was most important, but hallucinated images of what was in the outside world. The infant's mind was torn in the 'paranoid-schizoid position', Klein argued, between objects and part-objects that gave material sustenance and satisfaction, with the 'good breast' fitting the bill, and horrifying persecutory phantasies of dismemberment by the 'bad breast', that which was unavailable, withdrawn, frustrating.

Such phantasies, which Kleinians insist on spelling with 'ph' rather than 'f' to remind us that they are unconscious, whirl around the mind as if it were a container, with instincts as the drivers, real base 'instincts', a term Klein herself insisted upon, knowing well the debates over the translation of *Trieb* as 'drive' into the English language. I taught this approach as a theory of personality at Manchester Polytechnic to disbelieving psychology students, one of whom asked me after a lecture how the infant knew which was the good and which was the bad breast. It was a question that replicated what Klein and her followers called 'splitting', in which qualities of the world are rendered into separate objects of perception and then loved or hated, experienced as loving or hating. Most of the time the infant hated, was envious; it wanted, Klein said, to scoop out the insides of the mother to attack the bad and obtain the good. When she said the infant wanted to attack the father's penis from inside the mother, she really meant penis, not a symbolic phallus.

The depressive position into which a patient in analysis might move, a position in which they might make 'reparation' for the hatred they directed at the bad breast when they realise it is very same object that they loved and that was offered to them as a sign of love, was itself precarious. The depressive position had to be fought for after working through permutations of phantasy in the transference relationship with their analyst. Perhaps it was precisely because Klein's description was so categorical, a strict grid, itself paranoid-schizoid we might say, that it was taken up in the sociology of work and in nursing.

Elliott Jaques, a Canadian sociologist who worked with Melanie Klein, was one reference point for psychoanalytic sociology in Britain after the Second World War. Jaques had stayed on in London, after being assigned to help psychiatrists in the War Office Selection Boards during the war, and in 1951 published *The Changing Culture of a Factory*, in which splitting and projection – the placing of instinctual processes in others so that they would then be experienced as coming from those others rather than from inside oneself – were key concepts. Trades union negotiators who saw management as persecutory, for example, could then be enjoined to move from their paranoid-schizoid position to a depressive position in which they would appreciate the good along with the bad and participate in negotiations in better spirit. Jaques repudiated this Kleinian approach after founding a new school of social sciences at what became Brunel University of West London in the 1960s, so his work was treated by Kleinian sociologists as a good historical reference point but not as a perfect model for what they wanted to develop.

More influential still, and less obviously reactionary politically, was the work of Isabel Menzies Lyth, who had a background in experimental psychology in Scotland before coming to London to work in the War Office Selection Boards, carry out research on nurse training guided by Elliott Jaques, and then train as a Kleinian psychoanalyst. It was the nurse-training research that made Menzies Lyth's name among the Kleinian sociologists in a much-cited 1959 study, first published in the Tavistock Institute journal *Human Relations*, titled 'The functioning of social systems as a defence against anxiety'. While the Jaques research on factories riled some students who wanted, quite rightly, to know what the consequences of his reductionist diagnosis of splitting and projection would be for trades union resistance to real exploitation at work, the Menzies Lyth study chimed with the experience of almost every student who had encountered the care system, either as trainee nurses or as other kinds of carers in and around hospitals.

Hospitals are wellsprings of anxiety, with nurses as well as patients confronted with pain and mortality. For trainee nurses the social system of the hospital – the network of often inexplicable rules that hold life in place – is a means for coping with this anxiety. The thought that these patients might die, and that some of them will certainly die, is mobilised by the hospital context and then defended against. This is why human beings are turned into objects, not love objects in a directly psychoanalytic sense of the term, but as patients treated as numbers and tasks. Menzies Lyth notes the function of such practices as referring to 'the liver in bed 10' instead of the name of the patient, or waking patients up to give them their sleeping pills at a set time. The unthinkable is erased by such social systems, which run through the health service as a place of permanent personal threat. We knew in Manchester, for example, that the first designs for the new Manchester Royal Infirmary across the road from the site of our polytechnic did not include space for a mortuary. Menzies Lyth provided at least some initial diagnoses for thinking and working through why that may have happened, why those working in hospitals could not bear to think that people sometimes die there.

Beyond

The Elliott Jaques and Isabel Menzies Lyth studies laid the bedrock of British Kleinian sociology. The sociology part of the equation was no guarantee that their use of psychoanalysis would be progressive, that it would be any better than simplistic psychological explanations of political processes. We could see very clearly in the case of Jaques' work that reduction to the sociological level could screen out structural social inequalities and power relations just as efficiently as psychology usually did, and Menzies Lyth had nothing to say about the broader social context, in which hospitals come to function as the site of dread of death, often sealed off from the community, and with nursing hierarchies leaving apprentices overworked and unable to question what they are told.

An exception to this picture, someone who contrasted with the British tradition approach but who contributed to it a more explicit political sociology, was the US-based psychoanalyst Joel Kovel. His work fed into the British psychoanalytic debates. Kovel, who was also at the 1987 Psychoanalysis and Public Sphere conference, had trained as an IPA psychoanalyst in the US, but always grounded his writing in a social context. I set his 1976 book *A Complete Guide to Therapy: From*

Psychoanalysis to Behaviour Modification as required reading for my counselling option; he mentioned in the introduction to the book that he had started off as a Reichian, concerned with radical social change, but warned the reader about his 'therapeutic conservativism'. He had been most unhappy with the publisher insisting on a change of title from the original, more accurate 'Critical Guide to Therapy' that he had been writing to, and grumbled about the change.

Kovel took an explicitly more radical tack in his 1983 book *Against the State of Nuclear Terror*, and these were ideas popularised in a documentary directed by Denis Postle and screened on Channel 4 in a series called 'Crucible: Science in Society'. Channel 4 was the fourth television channel to broadcast in the UK in the 1980s, and quickly gained a reputation for experimental and politically-progressive programming. The Crucible series was run by Bob Young, the radical historian of science who had edited *Radical Science Journal* and who was now co-organising the 1987 NELP conference. 'Radical Science', as Bob Young would have it, was an approach to empirical inquiry and knowledge production that explored how the cultural-political preoccupations of cultures, institutions and research teams led to certain kinds of questions being asked about the nature of the world and human beings. It was an approach to science that was, in some sense of the term, 'social constructionist'. He had argued in a classic article ten years before, published in *Radical Science Journal*, that 'science *is* social relations', but he also wanted to show how the 'social constructions' of the world, which scientists circulated among themselves and in the popularisation of their discoveries, were grounded in material structures. He wrote as a Marxist. At least, that's how I read him.

Although Joel Kovel was a psychoanalyst, he became dissatisfied with the way his work in the clinic dealt with social problems such as alienation and racism – as if they were a result of individual childhood conflicts. His 1988 *White Racism* extended the work of revolutionary psychiatrist and activist Frantz Fanon. In his 1981 book *The Age of Desire*, Kovel had presented fictionalised 'case histories', which showed how the symptoms that afflicted these individuals' lives were a reflection of deeper problems in capitalist society. That book made public one stage in Kovel's personal journey to Marxism. In his 1983 *Against the State of Nuclear Terror* and the Channel 4 documentary, he was concerned with what he called 'technocracy', the forms of power that separated people from each other and created states of fear, which psychologists and psychoanalysts then encountered in the clinic. The documentary included footage of Kovel in 'cooperative inquiry' groups, which were at once therapeutic spaces to reflect on this sense of fear and threat and at the same time designed to mobilise people so they could take collective action against the nuclear state that created and maintained those psychologically-paralysing feelings.

I used this book and video in my teaching. Kovel's argument was double-edged. On the one hand it used bits of psychology, psychoanalytic descriptions of 'defences' that people used to shield themselves from feelings of threat, and on the other hand it drew attention to the limits of seeing those defences as only operating at the level of the individual. Here it connected with Menzies Lyth's social-psychoanalytic analysis of hospitals as social systems that provoked and contained anxiety. For Kovel, the 'state' of nuclear terror referred to the political entities set against each other in the logic of 'Mutually Assured Destruction', and they relied on passive, frightened acceptance by their populations. This was a political problem that also relayed forms of social 'defence' into each individual, so that they experienced themselves as if they were little 'states' under threat, suspicious of other people.

This was more immediately useful than the Lacanian work I encountered when I arrived in Manchester, the leader of the post-structuralists at that time being Antony Easthope, a literary theorist who taught cultural studies at Manchester Polytechnic. Easthope was a one-time Marxist who had been an active member of the Independent Labour Party, and who referred to his time in Marx and Freud reading groups as his 'long march through the institutions', a deliberate reference to Mao's long march before the 1949 revolution in China. With Rob Lapsley and Mike Westlake, he was responsible for inducting generations of leftist academics into post-structuralism and postmodernism in evening classes in Manchester in the 1980s. Easthope was an endearing and infuriating figure, smoking a cigar at you while he repeated his own particular version of Lacan's dictum that you should not give ground relative to your desire – it does not mean you should enact everything you desire – whisking you back to his house in Didsbury in time to watch his favourite film review programme so you could watch him argue with Barry Norman, the presenter.

Easthope's engagement with psychoanalysis also illustrated how easy it was to slide from the quite surreal and subversive aspects of a Freudian or Lacanian approach to culture into psychology, how easy it was to turn it into psychology. He knew well that Freud should be read with an eye to the literary rhetorical aspects of the text, and once told a meeting we invited him to, for example, that while there were no jokes in the standard medical text *Gray's Anatomy*, you would find in Freud the delightful idea that men wore ties because they could at last decide on the length and colour of the thing that dangled from their bodies. There are many more jokes in Freud, he said. Easthope would often turn up with a question about something he had read in Freud or Lacan, wanting to know what experimental research study he might read and cite to support it. He sometimes looked at me as if I was holding this knowledge back and refusing out of laziness or spite, when I tried to explain why a psychological account of what was going on would have the opposite effect from the one he was hoping for, and eventually he gave up asking.

Easthope's intervention at a meeting organised by Psychologists for Peace in Manchester was fairly typical. This was for a network that was focusing on the question of nuclear threat and cautiously taking up some of Joel Kovel's ideas, while keeping the political critique of the nuclear state out of the picture. Easthope turned up and claimed that those involved were fascinated with death; the death instinct underpinned pious calls for 'peace', he said, just as involvement in organisations protesting against torture was driven by an unconscious desire to know more about torture. He did in this, at least, express something of the other side of the use of psychoanalysis, the danger that this kind of theory could just as quickly cut back against those of us who wanted it to be a progressive alternative to mainstream psychology.

The Psychologists for Peace people themselves very tentatively used some psychoanalytic ideas about 'defence mechanisms' that people might use to protect themselves against feelings of threat, but they wanted to keep scientific psychology in command. They didn't want to open the Pandora's box of the unconscious and so threaten to unravel the version of the 'rational unitary subject' that they were committed to. They had managed to get the British Psychological Society to publish their book on the 'psychological aspects' of nuclear war on the understanding that it was reasoned scientific debate that would enable us to understand that threat, and that every individual involved should be treated as a reasoning holistic person. Many of those involved were deeply committed to exactly the kind of humanistic psychology that the radical Foucauldian psychoanalytic book *Changing the Subject* excoriated.

Antony Easthope's comments at our conference in Manchester realised their worst fears and suspicions about where psychoanalysis would lead. Those debates also opened a window on traditions of 'radical psychology' that had been around for many years before *Changing the Subject*, well-meaning attempts to bring psychological expertise to bear on social policy, to persuade politicians not to escalate nuclear conflict. On the one hand, Easthope's comments were an antidote to the rather hopeless expectation that politicians would listen to psychologists, or psychoanalysts for that matter. On the other hand, Joel Kovel's active engagement with these questions was a more constructive, less cynical response. The 'affinity groups' Kovel called for in his book *Against the State of Nuclear Terror* were part of a grass-roots mobilisation of people to deal with threat, and a challenge to the institutions that were responsible for escalating that threat.

Beneath

This brings us to Psychoanalysis and the Public Sphere in 1987. I was disappointed when Kovel said, in one session of the conference, that the most important thing for someone wanting to use psychoanalysis for radical purposes was to go and get a good training in which the clinical and theoretical rigour was of overriding importance. I could see no good reason why people should be funnelled into training if they wanted to do something radical with psychoanalysis, and the suggestion that a traditional training would be of help seemed ludicrous. It would surely just draw radicals closer to a psychoanalytic world view, a reactionary one. I saw Kovel's comment as sidestepping the question of politics, and as turning psychoanalysis into a respectable clinical practice, an approach that effectively put the radical tradition of people like Wilhelm Reich aside. I wondered if psychoanalysis in practice is often not as radical as its followers would like to believe, and it often functions as a kind of therapeutic consolation, enabling people to get along with their lives in impossible circumstances, encouraging people to live with the world as it is instead of changing it.

It became very clear in the two days at NELP that the conference was Bob Young's baby, or, at least, one of his babies, nurtured alongside his psychoanalytic firstborn, the journal *Free Associations*, which had begun publication three years before. The birth of *Free Associations* was told as a story of trauma, a psychoanalytic account of a political project that replicated the psychoanalytic language it was dedicated to promoting. Bob Young, the editor and publisher, would say as much himself, a purveyor of gossip that he especially enjoyed when he was the main protagonist. He had been in the same class at Yale as Joel Kovel and the social constructionist psychologist Ken Gergen. Here, Bob's story was that the Crucible: Science in Society Channel 4 television series, into which he poured all his energy as the conduit for ideas he had been developing in his *Radical Science Journal*, hit the buffers in 1983. That was the year of Margaret Thatcher's triumphant electoral victory, a second term of office following the Falklands War, and now she was determined to settle scores with cultural institutions like Channel 4 that were viewed as being broadly on the left, a thorn in her side during her first term. The new commissioning editor had been one of Thatcher's speech-writers during the election and told Young so during a phone call before informing him that the Crucible series was finished. Young went into shock, and then into analysis, Kleinian psychoanalysis, very soon after setting up Free Association Books and its house journal *Free Associations*, financial liabilities that would eventually necessitate remortgaging his house in Freegrove Road in north London. At Free Association Books, he republished classics in psychoanalysis that he saw as being in some sense 'radical', including Menzies Lyth's work as *Containing Anxiety in Institutions*.

Bob Young was very Kleinian, a big man with strong black-rimmed glasses and a black-and-red checked shirt and braces. He liked to say he was from Dallas, Texas, and boom this bit of biographical information out from the centre of the room, usually as a preface to something provocative, sometimes outrageous. As for any true Kleinian, there was for him, first and foremost, violence inside the psyche, the death instinct, and it was no good pretending that it, the war within, was not there.

I was living in Kentish Town in north London at that time, and my then-partner was outraged when our son Ben came home one day in 1984 from the Young house with a wooden gun Bob had lashed together for the boys, breaking, and probably deliberately defying, the rule against violent toys in our home. I was keeping my distance from psychoanalysis then, concerned that it was effectively part of the 'psy' complex, complicit in adjusting people to society rather than enabling them to challenge it. I said this to the child psychoanalyst Margot Waddell, Bob's then-partner, on their doorstep one day when I was delivering something back to her house, not the wooden gun, and she looked at me pityingly. I guessed she would have a reason in mind for my resistance to psychoanalysis, and I think she knew I knew this. The difference between us was awkward and irresolvable, and still unresolved when I turned up at the NELP jamboree three years on.

It turned out that the 'my wife' comment by Mike Rustin at the beginning of the conference unwittingly spoke to and of a fractious context behind the scenes at

Free Associations. The founding premise of the journal was that British psychoanalysis, which is primarily Kleinian alongside what was viewed as softer-core object-relations theory, was politically progressive, to the left or left of centre. That phrase, 'free association' spoke to psychoanalysts, for whom it named the fundamental technical rule of the clinic – for the analysand to say everything that came to mind however irrelevant, stupid or unpleasant – but also signalled a link to the political tradition in which it is, as Marx has it, an association in which the free development of each is the condition for the free development of all.

Free Associations would thus function as a forum to draw the psychoanalysts even further to the left, perhaps even to radicalise the main institutions, most importantly the British Psychoanalytical Society and its training wing, the Institute of Psychoanalysis. There were no Lacanians involved in this, and they would not have been welcome. Bob Young had bigger fish to fry. The leading Kleinian psychoanalyst in Britain, Hanna Segal, for example, had been co-founder of Psychoanalysts Against Nuclear Warfare, and this was another green light for the Free Associations project.

The most burning issue at the Psychoanalysis and the Public Sphere conference in 1987, however, was not nuclear war but the exclusion of lesbians and gay men from IPA training in Britain, an issue that went to the heart of psychoanalytic theories of sexuality and cut at the limits of most practitioners' liberalism, let alone left and feminist practice in the psychoanalytic institutions. A couple of years before, two psychoanalytic psychotherapists, Noreen O'Connor and Joanna Ryan had brought out with Virago, a feminist publisher, *Wild Desires and Mistaken Identities: Lesbianism and Psychoanalysis*, which lifted the lid on the way that the Institute of Psychoanalysis in London routinely turned away intending candidates on the basis that they had unresolved issues to do with their sexuality.

There were psychoanalysts trained at the Institute who came out to their colleagues only after they qualified, but this pointed to an even deeper, more pernicious problem with the training. Because the psychoanalyst in a 'training analysis' was expected to report on the progress of the candidate to the training committee, the odds were that in some cases the candidates were, rather incredibly, keeping quiet about that aspect of their sexuality. Noreen and Joanna were at the conference to convene a session on the question, but there was evident puzzlement among some of the analysts about why this was an issue. The session was packed. Christoph Hering, a psychotherapist and NELP lecturer, commented during the session that in all the years of his practice he had never encountered anyone who was gay. The incredulity and resentment was palpable, and the charged atmosphere in this session spilled out, to and from other sessions. This is "impossible", the feminist psychoanalytic scholar Amal Treacher muttered to me in a tea break, referring to the behaviour of some of the men.

Bob Young brought the Frankfurt School critique of the assumed opposition between culture and nature to life at the conference. This is a split bound up with the Cartesian dualist division between mind and body, something so relevant to psychoanalysis, to the historical conditions of possibility, for it to take as a social and clinical practice. Responding to talk among the conference-goers about what was 'natural', Bob drew attention to the way they all-too-often idealised nature, romanticised it – and that the commodification of nature could be seen in the lotions and potions from places like the Body Shop that they frequented. There was nervous laughter as he said, "I know, I've seen inside your bathrooms." He was on form. It was also a reminder that 'free association' as such is actually impossible in psychoanalysis, and it is a mistake to believe that you can really say everything, make the unconscious conscious. It is the failure to free associate – the hesitations, ellipses and slips that reveal something of the process by which things are kept unconscious – that is of interest to psychoanalysis.

A South African white psychotherapist referred in another session to black students as being like children, which, in albeit muted therapeutic form, led Farhad Dalal and me to respond as energetically as we felt able. We complained, and Barry Richards, a clinical psychologist at NELP who was, along with Mike Rustin, the main link for Free Associations to hold the conference, told us that this was obviously for all of us a "difficult, painful issue". The South African was astonished that we should object, telling us that we misunderstood, and that even when they were behaving in an infantile violent way he loved black people like his own children. Richards' response was of a piece with the idea that those who were protesting against injustice should also tolerate pain, and, it seemed to me, should accept that some things could not be changed. He rehearsed this line in a fierce debate with Joel Kovel in the journal *Radical Philosophy*, a conservative response to political resistance that was also spun out at great length in a book by Ian Craib called *The Importance of Disappointment*, one that was popular with therapists busy abandoning their previous leftist history and who wanted to justify this step to themselves.

Psychoanalysis in the British tradition was very practised at infantilising those who protested against exploitation, like the factory workers in the Jaques study, or those who complained about bad behaviour, like some of us who were reminded that we should know that things are difficult and painful, and be prepared to move on from paranoid-schizoid splitting into good and bad, move on to a reparative relationship to our objects of love and hate, to the depressive position. It was depressing that the Institution of Psychoanalysis was itself operating as a social system to defend itself against the anxiety that it provoked. Perhaps I was more anxious now that I was evidently no longer completely outside of all this, but getting drawn into it.

6

CONVERSATIONS

Taking care of health

Psychoanalysis in social theory is all well and good, but I was also beginning to be more interested in how it worked out in practice, and how to make sense of competing approaches to psychotherapy in the British National Health Service. We can see here how psychoanalytic ideas have needed to adapt themselves to health institutions in order to survive. Bit by bit, by engaging more with the theory and exploring how it worked from the inside, and lured in further by the idea that I could be an amateur anthropologist in the strange world of psychoanalytic psychotherapy, I was getting drawn into clinical work.

Acting

It was, I admit, rather fraudulent of me to teach counselling approaches in the final year of an undergraduate degree course when I had no first-hand experience of counselling or psychotherapy. I knew this was not unusual. Most colleagues around me, and in other institutions, taught about cognitive-behavioural and humanistic approaches as well as about the shortcomings of Freudian psychoanalysis, without ever having been consumers of therapy, let alone having undergone practical clinical training. This was acceptable in psychology departments that were wedded to the model of the 'scientist-practitioner' in clinical psychology, a model that had been promoted since the end of the Second World War by Hans Eysenck, based at the Institute of Psychiatry in Denmark Hill, south London. There was something rotten about this. There was no requirement that clinical psychologists should undergo therapy themselves as part of their training; instead they did things to other people, clients, patients, who were assumed to be different from them.

Even some of the more humanistic counselling organisations that sent guest speakers to talk about their service into Manchester Polytechnic still worked on the assumption that there was a difference between the healthy experts and their sick clientele. I heard from students who worked as volunteers and then wanted to work full-time in such organisations, for example, that they were even sometimes told that they should not talk about having been service users themselves at interview. The versions of psychoanalysis that were taught on most academic programmes, whether psychology or film theory, were so cut off from clinical practice that the idea that people still free-associated, or lay on couches while they did so, seemed outlandish to students, even to some of the lecturers. I had plenty of excuses to avoid therapeutic practice while I taught psychoanalytic theory, but it still felt bad, wrong. And, in addition to my guilt at this bad faith – the sense that I was merely acting the part, while extolling the benefits of different models of therapy or picking holes in them, the sense of banal fraudulence that many academics feel in the face of allied professionals – I was curious. There were other worlds I knew little about, should have done, wanted to, other worlds that I was excluded from.

The next best thing to visiting such other worlds, second-best imaginative exploration in the science-fiction paperbacks and US-American superhero comic-books brought into our house by my stepfather and his friends, was the annual Festival of Mind Body Spirit, which I had plundered for wacky 'New Age' cult literature since its first London event in 1977. Evangelists from different groups devoted to herb and crystal cures or, better, hidden cosmologies, would hawk their wares from behind stalls, and be eager to induct you into their world view. One of my favourites at these events was the Aetherius Society, which, relayed through Dr George King messages from Mars about the dangers of nuclear war on this planet. I was an amateur anthropologist at these events, and knew how to show a measure of guarded interest, interest enough to get these folk to open up. I listened well, and loved hearing about the direct-contact shamans had with alternate realities, about contact with other planets and the conspiracies that prevented the messages from other civilisations being heard by all.

I loved that these people believed these things fervently enough to give their lives to strange causes, to theories about the nature of the universe, theories that were patently untrue but that had some kind of internal coherence, that made sense to those who traced their way around their own chosen hermetic system of knowledge. Something of these parallel worlds attracted me to psychology, a discipline I never bought into on its own terms. Its power to enforce ways of speaking about the mind troubled me, and fascinated me, and I wanted to know how it worked from the inside. But experimental psychology's mechanistic and limited accounts of what went on inside the head began to pall and the wondrous lifeworlds of psychotherapists began to function in their place, as even more amazing stories about selves and social relationships began to draw me in.

At the edge of the Psychology for Peace networks were psychoanalytic psychotherapists from the late Reichian tradition who participated in groups, exploring the threat of war that figured in the Joel Kovel documentary *Against the State of Nuclear Terror*. By 'late Reichian', I mean the more bizarre Reich who, towards the end of his life, elaborated a theory of 'Orgone energy'. Orgone is a bluish-tinged pulsing life force that could, he believed, be seen in the sky and released from the clouds. Kate Bush's music video 'Cloudbusting', released in 1985, was about this force. These therapists took up the notion of 'character armour' Reich had described in his earlier psychoanalytic writings, but, instead of dealing with it through a classical Freudian 'talking cure', went straight to the body to deal with it through 'bodywork', massage and suchlike. I visited one of the groups in London.

My experience of making contact with the post-Reichians was about as satisfying as when I tried to get access to the Arbours Association house, one of the R. D. Laing radical psychiatry communities, when I was asked how I was going to fund my time there, or when I tried wangle a trip to Cuba to defend the revolution a couple of years earlier at the Cuban Embassy. They were as puzzled by my request as I was clueless about what it entailed. I eventually settled for a psychology degree in Plymouth instead. Anyway, back to the Reichians: one of the guys I recognised from the Kovel documentary was friendly but suspicious, and wanted to know what I could offer. Nothing, of course, this would go nowhere. Perhaps it was also clear that I was window-shopping, in Mind Body Spirit customer mode. Then I heard that there was an opening in a therapy group in the Manchester Royal Infirmary, the MRI psychiatry department across the road from our campus of Manchester Polytechnic. It was one of the off-the-wall approaches described in the wacky left-field book *Innovative Therapy in Britain,* Jacob Moreno's psychodrama.

There was another autobiographical tributary to this channel into psychodrama and psychotherapeutic practice. Alongside guilt at not having experienced what I was describing in my teaching, my haunted fraudulent play-acting, and my enjoyment at anthropological journeys into weird world views, my voyeuristic eavesdropping, I did once want to be an actor. My mother and stepfather took it seriously. I was enrolled in Rose Bruford College acting classes on Saturdays while I was in primary school, but the double bus journey to Sidcup in south London was a pain, and I lost heart. Standing up in front of the lecture class was a poor substitute, but, then, that's what substitutes and sublimation are all about, poor and manageable alternatives to what presents itself in fantasy as star billing somewhere else.

A group tears me in two. On the one hand it is an opportunity to perform in front of others, with the separation between actor and their audience also providing some distance, some protection. I have always preferred lectures to seminars or the small groups of tutorials. On the other hand, a group demands considerate, measured participation, letting others speak too, sharing the attention, which can be irritating, bordering on outright jealousy.

Jacob Moreno, like Reich, took a shortcut to action. Instead of meticulously tracing through the detours of speech, psychodrama was a chance to directly re-enact past relationships as they had been and as they could have been. Moreno had encountered Freud at the beginning of the century in Vienna before he, Moreno, moved to the US, but quickly diverged from a psychoanalytic approach, developing instead a particular form of therapy from his improvisational dramatic experiments in a 'Theatre of Spontaneity', and back-writing an alternative theory of the self into the practice. This psychodrama, Moreno claimed, was therapy in the world and, as for Reich but without the organised communist politics, was vaunted as a more progressive, engaged form of therapy, a reason some leftists in the therapy world are attracted to it.

Psychodrama was not really in the world, of course, but on stage; it staged symptomatic and spontaneous behaviour in order to notice what was going on. So, it was group work instead of one-to-one individual therapy, with an often-implicit radical-political gloss to justify that. It claimed to work with spontaneity and reflection rather than structured speech; it involved action, rather than attending to what could not be said in the Freudian clinic's always doomed attempt to free associate, it was faster perhaps. For someone impatient to get going in therapy after I had spent so much time avoiding it, this was perfect. I joined a new group in July 1989.

The group facilitators, Stuart and Jan, were psychiatric nurses at the MRI. We met for our two-hour psychodrama group in the conference room in Rawnsley Building, a multi-coloured window-frame, Lego-block part of the psychiatric inpatient and outpatient facility that seemed designed to infantilise the residents. We were effectively outpatients, but, it became clear, the 'normal' ones, shut off from the wards by locked doors with reinforced wire-strip glass. This was a staff group, and I got into it by virtue of teaching across the road, the only lecturer among nurses and support workers. Stuart, bearded, with the demeanour of the jolly provocateur, wore a Robinson's jam golliwog enamel badge in his lapel, and clearly enjoyed being challenged over this, so I didn't react. Jan was an efficient guide to the process and took notes that, occasionally, we would be invited to see being written up after the session, when they trusted us more, part of staff training for some of the participants. Psychiatric nursing staff were there not only to experience the group but also to be on track to run such a group themselves, which was the way of much informal internal education in the health service, cheaper apprenticeship through practice. This was what would enable me, too, to get access to the service without certificated training.

We would rotate our turn to play out a concern from our lives, which in the early sessions of the six-month life of the group would be such things as a hectoring supervisor who was difficult to say no to, or stress at work with a mounting burden of tasks. In later sessions we burrowed down a little deeper and earlier to family relationships – difficult, distant or overprotective parents or competitive siblings. This was always where we were heading, and the stage was set very early on for a reframing in the setting-up of the psychodrama, followed by our interpretations of what was going on, which focused attention on what we had learned about who we were and how we should experience our own families.

In one early session, for example, tables and chairs and other members of the group were arranged around and above me to depict the increasing workload I was dealing with across the road in the Polytechnic. Stuart and Jan encouraged me to build into the picture a figure who would be reaching in to hold my hand and give me comfort and strength. Afterwards the other group members were quick to interpret this figure as my mother. This set the scene for a further psychodrama, some weeks later, when it was my turn again: the solution to my experience of isolation in one context was again remedied by bringing in an avatar of my mother, who I was expected to hug. Quite a few of the scenarios did eventually resolve themselves into the enactment of an embrace with a parental figure. The denouement of these improvised dramatic scenes started to be predictable, and when the group ended I felt glad of the experience and glad it was over.

Speaking

While I was participating in the psychodrama group at MRI, I also attended Monday morning seminars at the local National Health Service psychotherapy service at Gaskell House. It was there that I met Bob Hobson, the guiding light or, as one of the junior psychiatrists once put it, the 'beating heart' of psychoanalytic approaches in Manchester psychotherapy.

Psychoanalysis had a much bigger impact in Britain in social and welfare services in the mid-twentieth century than in psychology as such – in the child guidance clinics and in the development of social work training, for example. There was a Freudian and post-Freudian wave in institutionalised welfare provision after the Second World War, in which John Bowlby was important in shaping the way that practitioners thought about the legacy of 'attachment' of infant to mother, worrying about the effect of insecure or disorganised attachment when women were drafted into armaments factories, and encouraging them to return to the home when the war was over. Bowlby helped popularise psychoanalytic ideas, as did Donald Winnicott after the war, through BBC radio broadcasts mainly aimed at women as mothers, and this popularisation was made possible, in part, by a softening bordering on banalisation of those ideas.

The British Psychoanalytical Society during the war had been riven by internal disputes, fuelled by the arrival of Melanie Klein in Britain in the 1920s and the formation of a group inside the society around her ideas, a group that then conflicted with the Freuds, with Sigmund and daughter Anna when they arrived in the late 1930s as refugees from Nazism. The internal disputes known as the 'Controversial Discussions' revolved around the role of internal, unconscious phantasy versus actual experience of object relations by the infant under the care of its mother. The main protagonists, Mrs Klein and Ms Freud, as well as many of their most prominent supporters, were women, but this war inside the British Psychoanalytical Society was eventually resolved by a so-called 'Gentleman's Agreement' in which there would be separate educational regimes at the Society's training wing, the Institute of Psychoanalysis. For a half-century since, the Institute (and the Society) was effectively divided into three groups: the Anna Freudians, the Kleinians, and a so-called 'Middle Group' of independents, of which Bowlby and Winnicott were the most well-known in the outside world. These three strands of work comprise the IPA in the British tradition.

While the Anna Freudians in the B Group were closest to the US-American ego-psychologists, emphasising the role of adaptive and maladaptive 'defence mechanisms' that buttressed the ego as the thinking, reasoning centre of the mind, the independent psychoanalysts in the Middle Group also followed a parallel track of work, theorising what would make for productive thought and healthy relationships. They set themselves against the A-Group Kleinians who saw the interior of the psyche as what one analyst, Edward Glover, referred to as a combination of a butcher's shop, a public lavatory under shell fire and a post mortem room. The independents were responsible for some of the most far-reaching revisions of Freudian theory, including attention to the 'containing' role of the psychoanalyst who would replicate a good-enough mothering environment. One of Britain's most influential feminists, Juliet Mitchell, was to train at the Institute and participate in the Middle Group.

These psychoanalysts did not really have the power to push through government policies concerning employment of women, but the psychoanalysts were pushing to be heard, and some pockets of the new National Health Service, at the Tavistock Clinic for example, fell under their influence. In different parts of the country, different psychoanalytic currents of work that reflected these debates in the British Psychoanalytical Society were able to find a home on condition that the analysts adapt their practice to the public welfare provision ethos of the NHS and, of course, to budget-conscious management structures. Group work was one way of cutting costs, and another was training for medical practitioners in the rudiments of psychotherapy, which, in Manchester under the auspices of Bob Hobson, meant turning a generation of psychiatrists towards the idea of listening to their clients instead of merely diagnosing their complaints and dishing out medication.

This Bob, Bob Hobson, a craggy, grey, wavy-haired elderly gentleman, hesitant, stuttering in a way that was often replicated by the junior staff he supervised, was a lapsed Jungian analyst. We, particularly those of us interested in Freudian and post-Freudian theories, and especially those of us who disliked the 'rational unitary subject', disliked Jungians. John Churcher, an academic colleague who was teaching up the road at the University of Manchester, used to tell his students, if they asked about Jung, that this non-Freudian work made him feel sick. Then, of course, the students would rush to the library and dig out all the books they could find about Jung's 'analytical psychology' and the ideas would emerge, the return of the repressed, in essays and exam answers.

We disliked Jungian analytical psychology not only because Jung stayed as head of the German Medical Society for Psychotherapy after the Nazis took power and wrote some antisemitic things that delighted his new masters, but also because, as for other psychologists, the aim of 'analysis' in that tradition was to heal the split between conscious and personal unconscious, restoring the self to a wholesome unity in what he called 'individuation'. This is not psychoanalysis. Bob Hobson was not only a lapsed Jungian, however, having resigned his membership of the Society for Analytical Psychology, but openly critical, developing instead an approach to therapy that was known as the 'conversational model'. It was this conversational model that became influential on a generation of therapists and psychiatrists in the NHS in Manchester.

The Monday morning group at Gaskell House would discuss individual client work, but also novels and films, putting different kinds of psychoanalytic ideas to work on popular culture. That's something I became more interested in, too, for it seemed to me that psychoanalytic ideas were powerful not only because they worked in the clinic, but also because they circulated through our culture, encouraging people to speak and then think about themselves in line with the theories. We knew what 'projection' was in psychoanalysis, the placing of an unwanted idea in another person and experiencing it as coming from them instead of from within ourselves, and we knew that Kleinians had added to this the idea of 'identification', the way in which we make ourselves at one with someone or with an idea, make it part of ourselves. Psychiatric nurse and therapist, Lisa Herzog, often reminded us of the internal psychic violence Mrs Klein was so adept at describing. Lisa would refer to nurses 'twisting the drip' at a bedside to cause pain as, of course, unconscious hostility to their patients. The Kleinian term 'projective identification' then takes us into a quite different, more frightening world, in which someone is thought to be able to actually project a thought or feeling into another so that the other thinks or feels what has been projected into them.

In one Monday morning session, Hobson claimed to have heard another member of the group say something that they then denied saying, to which he deferred before murmuring that it must have been a 'projective slip', that is, with the implication that there must be something going on between the two of them or in the group that led him to hear it as a slip. I found this fascinating; it was as if these people were living out a particular version of psychoanalysis they were deeply attached to, experiencing at depth, within themselves, the phenomena they described. Participants would speak about 'transferences flying about the room' as if these relationships between patient and therapist had taken on a reality independent of them, in much the same way that, in medieval Britain, people believed that invisible spirits fired arrows into people to make them distressed or elated. There was no good reason to take psychoanalytic descriptions circulated in the Hobson group any more seriously than the claims by members of the Aetherius Society that their leader Dr George King had heard the voices of Martians one morning while he was doing the washing-up. We were once again in Mind Body Spirit territory in Gaskell House.

I gave a paper at one of the Monday morning seminars about the paranoiac fantasies of abduction and evisceration among those who claimed they had been interfered with by aliens. It was an example, I argued, not so much of how some of Melanie Klein's more lurid ideas about 'splitting' and 'projection' powered by the 'death instinct' might be applied, but of how those ideas were picked up and then played out by people faced with experiences they couldn't otherwise make sense of. Afterwards Bob Hobson asked me if I had ever had these kinds of feelings about events I couldn't make sense of, and I knew as I said it, that I gave the right answer when I said that yes I had.

Listening

The psychoanalytic frame worked for these people, and I suspected that it must also work as a frame for those in distress who were desperate enough to buy into it. A Kleinian or Winnicottian or, why not, Jungian, frame of reference must, for some people, provide as much comfort as believing in the existence of Martians. Dr George King's Aetherius Society would also be well able to explain such things, with the difference that a therapist working in one of those psychoanalytic frames could also maintain the frame as a containing place in which speculation about conspiracies and threats of different kinds could be mediated and ameliorated. I tussled with the question as to whether the psychoanalytic narratives I was hearing at Gaskell House and teaching about in the Poly were historically-specific constructions of self or universal, but decided that, if I wanted to know more about how they were constructed, I would need to suspend disbelief and explore them from the inside.

The Monday morning group was not deliberately designed to induct people into therapy, but it did eventually lead several of us outsiders to want to become insiders. Our participation in the group was a sign that we could talk the talk, and financial pressure on the NHS led the therapists in charge of the group to ask some of us whether we would be willing to see a patient in the service under supervision. The psychotherapy service manager, Alan Horne, a quietly-spoken, thoughtful presence on Monday mornings, posed the question about our involvement and invited us in to help out in the service.

It seems an extraordinarily unthinkable arrangement now. I had no training, had never worked as a counsellor, but I would be allowed to take on a patient. "It is more like counselling," Frank Margison, who was clinical director at Gaskell House, said in my interview for an honorary appointment in November 1991, "and we are in a catchment area that includes a lot of academics so we don't have as detailed monitoring of patient details." Here is another Frank, psychoanalytic Frank. So, I thought, this means that middle-class people will have a more confidential service. To get onto the waiting lists, referred from their family doctor or from an outpatient service, there is already a filtering out of those who do not already have some notion that there is something unconscious to them, what is usually referred to in the NHS psychotherapy services as 'psychological mindedness'. Psychotherapy patients are invariably PLU, People Like Us – and so it was when my first patient, Martin, was eventually selected eighteen months later from the waiting list for an eighteen-month once-weekly stretch of therapy.

I have jumbled details from different patients in this book, of course, and not simply changed their names. I had already consumed tales of psychotherapy, from the entirely fictionalised case histories in Joel Kovel's *Age of Desire* to the stranger-than-fiction early bestseller, *The Fifty-Minute Hour* by Robert Lindner, first published in 1955 in the US and republished in 1986 by Free Association Books. Lindner's 'true psychoanalytic tales', as the subtitle has it, sold over a million and a half copies in the 1950s, and it was influential in the popularising of psychoanalysis. The final tale of the mad scientist in 'The Jet-Propelled Couch' invited much speculation as to the real identity of the patient. Irvin Yalom's *Love's Executioner*, which assiduously conceals who is who, I read while on holiday in Greece – the cover is spattered with blood from mosquitoes I dispatched along the way. Robert Akeret's *The Man Who Loved a Polar Bear* is not so careful: financially-pressed, Akeret looked up past patients and interviewed them about how much they had benefited from therapy with him – in one case Akeret had feigned a heart attack in the consulting room to evoke a caring response. How fascinating that terrible book is: was that really how it worked? Surely not. Bob Hobson's *Forms of Feeling* includes an account of being threatened by a patient with a gun, an account that drew some sharp criticism from readers who thought they could guess from clues in the text as to who that patient was.

I was, the letter from Alan Horne said, to be a 'psychotherapy trainee', and was put in a supervision group, with two other visiting therapists, run by Jean Rawsthorne who had a forbidding face and mountains of black frizzy hair that cascaded down her thin shoulders. The first eighteen months' supervision ran alongside the Monday morning groups as an informal apprentice training, during which I encountered Wilfred Bion's apt description of the consulting room as ideally containing two rather frightened people. My safety net, and that of the psychotherapy service, was a cassette recorder on which I was to record every session and bring the tape to weekly supervision. Martin would know this. From November 1993, for the next eighteen months, I would collect Martin from the downstairs waiting room, and then Geraldine the receptionist would open the door leading upstairs – a disconcertingly loud buzz would release the catch, a reminder that this was still a secure psychiatric service.

Frank Margison had warned us that the cassette recorder would never be forgotten during the sessions. It sat on the table as a silent witness, and we had watched Bob Hobson's 1970s training video for psychiatrists on the 'conversational model', in which Frank, in very wide-wing, jacket-lapels and long sideburns, introduced mock sessions and Hobson hesitantly drew attention to the recording equipment. There was no pretence that what was to be said was spontaneous; the architecture and the technology guided us along tracks of time that were as exigent as the rules of speech. I would be reminded by Jean each week that Martin, a much older man, who worked as an accountant in another part of the health service, wanted to get close to me. His referral for anxiety in relationships called for careful 'containment' of our time together, for my task of 'holding' him, and for explicit reminders to him when there were impending breaks in the therapy. I was told to interpret the transference, to always bring Martin's discussion of his difficulties with others to the way those difficulties were being re-enacted in relationship to me.

I learned to experience it in that way too. If Martin spoke about his dislike of quantification, of people being turned into objects in the accounting department where he worked, this was about me. I disliked quantitative approaches in my own department. If he talked about his love of science fiction films, this was me too, for so did I. I identified with him. It was as if he could read my mind. I had to resist the temptation to think that I could read his.

'Containment' and 'holding', therapeutic terms from Bion and Winnicott, signalled that this was a broadly object-relations approach, with Bob Hobson's 'conversational model' as an entrée into the psychoanalytic psychotherapeutic process proper. It was quite explicit in the supervision meetings that we were operating inside a structure that we had a responsibility to construct and maintain for the therapy to work, a structure that went well beyond the two individuals gazing at each other in the upstairs room at Gaskell House each week. Such a structure, a group element of the face-to-face meeting was implicitly present to Martin, implicit at least and sometimes quite evident. Perhaps he did want to get close to me, I reminded him enough times that this is what he wanted, and then we had to let go of this relationship. I felt sad. Martin brought me a flower in a pot wrapped up in gift paper in the final session. Would I have felt such a bond with a therapist if I was ever the patient? Now I would find out.

7

THERAPY

Closer encounters

As night follows day, my engagement with psychoanalysis as a therapist was followed by an engagement with it as a patient. I will describe three encounters with psychotherapists in order to trace out the process by which people find a psychoanalyst. It is not easy to find one when you need one, as you will see. It is not wise, of course, to believe what someone says about their failed encounters with others they have had such intimate relationships with, nor to believe what they say about their successful encounters. I had plenty of suppositions about psychoanalytic theory that framed what I was looking for in a practitioner, suppositions that are worked on, elaborated and worked through in the clinic as what psychoanalysts call 'transference'.

Frank

"You must meet Frank," said my colleague John. This is John Churcher en route to a train, training as an IPA Kleinian psychoanalyst at the Institute of Psychoanalysis. You have already met Frank. Frank Margison was the linchpin of the Gaskell House psychotherapy service, a key figure in the first generation of advocates of the conversational model as a way station to full-blown psychoanalytic provision in the NHS in Manchester, or the closest to it we could manage outside London. In addition to Bob Hobson, there was one other psychoanalyst, also with a Jungian background, Barbara Dick, who was based in north Manchester and Salford. Newcomers heard mutterings about historical differences between Gaskell House and the Red House over on the other side of the city, but it was difficult to get to the root of what the differences between those two National Health Service clinics were. There were no IPA psychoanalysts in Manchester, but quite a few psychoanalytic psychotherapists who were mostly clustered around the NWIDP, the North West Institute for

Dynamic Psychotherapy, an accredited training closely linked to Frank and the Hobson group and reliant on NHS-funded places for trainees. Trainees and graduates in and around the NWIDP deferred to the IPA's Institute of Psychoanalysis in London, agreeing to adopt the title 'psychoanalytic psychotherapist' rather than 'psychoanalyst', the preserve of the IPA, and then they jealously guarded their own preferred title against those lower down the pecking order, the psychodynamic counsellors.

Frank was a psychiatrist, as were many of those who attended the Gaskell House Monday morning seminars, the participant list filled out with psychiatric nurses, therapists and a few interlopers, academics. I'll tell you again now that I feared and disliked psychiatrists, and being buzzed through the internal security door to the upstairs rooms in Gaskell House always gave me a little kick, a kick of apprehension that I would be caught and sectioned, compulsorily detained. That I taught abnormal psychology at the Polytechnic and some classes for John at the university did not stop me from having the occasional nightmare about psychiatrists. Perhaps that teaching and involvement in mental health system survivor organisations further fuelled those kinds of persecutory fantasies. I had a long-running battle with colleagues who taught the biological bases of behaviour and psychopathology at the Polytechnic, and there another John, known to students as John Stallion, was sometimes keen to persuade me that mental illness was what it claimed to label, an illness in the brain.

I was removed from teaching on the psychopathology third-year option course because, that John said, I was having a bad influence on the students. I was exploring feminist arguments against psychiatry, the work of anti-colonial activist Frantz Fanon, and describing the work of the Hearing Voices support network, which had just set up shop in Manchester. I was making students sceptical about the scientific evidence for a biological cause of schizophrenia that John said. Exclusion from teaching on the course haunted me. I dreamt of it. In one recurring dream, I was in my office in 'E Block' at our campus, and, anxious that I had been locked into the building, I walked down the corridor late at night past John Stallion's office. His door was open, and I could see him strangling one of his male postgraduate students. Some romantic assignation between the two of them had turned bad, I thought. I ran back to my office, John chasing me down the corridor while shouting "I'll show you what real madness is." I barricaded my office door with a desk, and smashed the window, jumping through it just as John broke through, and I landed on the ground below impaled on his machine gun. Bad John.

John Churcher, good John the Kleinian, told me I should meet Frank Margison to discuss whether it would be possible for us three together to set up a 'psychoanalytic studies' postgraduate degree course jointly between Manchester Polytechnic, the University of Manchester and Gaskell House therapy service, perhaps involving the NWIDP: it would be a way of connecting academic qualifications with psychotherapy training. John had shown Frank the outline for my third-year option course, Psychoanalysis and Society, which first ran 1989–1990, and, John said, Frank liked the look of it. So we had meetings together at Gaskell House contemporaneous with the Monday Hobson group seminars, something that must have helped with the process of getting access to the service as honorary psychotherapist. Something else. Somewhere along the line in this process I decided that I wanted psychoanalysis, or something like it.

It wasn't that this was a prerequisite to working as a therapist in Gaskell House, but I did begin to sense that undergoing therapy oneself was part of the package, that it would not be right for me to subject someone else to therapy without having experience of it directly myself. In some ways this suspicion that I should go into therapy was payback for the scorn I had directed at clinical psychologists and psychiatrists who had nothing to do with the treatments they meted out to others. I had claimed that their professed scientific neutrality about the nature of distress was fraudulent, and now there were consequences of that claim – for me. The more time I spent with people who talked about therapy and, more to the point, the more they talked therapeutically about therapy, the more I felt torn between suspicion of this peculiar jargon about the nature of the self and a temptation to find out what it was like from the inside. Mind Body Spirit alternate realities again loomed large and they were working their way into the texture of my own life.

The social anthropologist Ernest Gellner writes about the way that people are inducted into Freudian and quasi-Freudian views of the world and theories about themselves in his 1985 book *The Psychoanalytic Movement: The Cunning of Unreason*. The issue for me was not that psychoanalytic theory was untested, which was one of the positivist Popper-like subsidiary claims of Gellner's book, but that psychoanalytic theory stepped in to fill a spiritual void in industrialised societies. Its power came from Freud and his followers' ability to anticipate objections to the theory as further evidence that psychoanalysis itself must be true, and so new recruits were won to the theory as they worked through and came to appreciate what their own resistance to Freudian ideas really signified. Claude Lévi-Strauss had made a similar claim in his 1949 paper 'The Sorcerer and His Magic', reprinted in his *Structural Anthropology* book; those who resisted would fall harder once they were drawn into the practice.

In some ways Gellner was rehashing some of the earlier objections to Freud, including Karl Kraus's well-known quip that psychoanalysis is the disease it pretends to cure, a nice dialectical reversal that true Freudians would themselves enjoy and even, on occasion, repeat and revel in. There was a rhetorical tangle in this claim that exemplified what Gellner was trying to draw attention to. But more than that, Gellner's argument tuned in to the way that devotees of psychoanalysis spoke about their internal resistances in line with psychoanalytic discourse, and so psychoanalytic discourse operated as a trap; once one started to speak it, one began to be inducted into a psychoanalytic vision of the world and the unconscious subjects who inhabited it.

A psychiatrist as a therapist would be scary, and I was sure I would not tell him about my psychiatric-phobic nightmares, but, then again, perhaps I would. I could think of no one else to ask for therapy – the usual predicament of someone searching for a psychoanalyst – and, apart from Bob Hobson, who was now quite old and so, I guessed, no longer taking on patients, Frank Margison was the obvious choice. One Thursday afternoon, in December 1992, while I was waiting to see my first NHS patient, I made an appointment with Frank to discuss this. He had a couch in the corner of his ground-floor office in Gaskell House.

Frank said no. He thought it would not be a good idea, given the other kinds of activities we were involved in together, the obvious answer. After I let the disappointment settle in and ruminated on his response for a while, it dawned on me how difficult it would be to speak to him both as patient and colleague. Even that frank 'no' sent a message that was way beyond the simple information it imparted. It was precisely because I felt that 'no' as rejection that I realised what it might be like to have him listen to me whining about my unconscious at one moment, wheedling for his love in the transference as a repetition in the clinic of past relationships to significant others, and then have a rational discussion about setting up a psychoanalytic studies course with John Churcher the next. I experienced it as a first lucky escape, when it was actually more the consequence of a clear, principled position that Frank took in response to my stupid, hasty request.

Ruth

A few weeks later I met Ruth Caro Salzberger in West Didsbury, the Hampstead of Manchester. This place, M20, could have been the psychoanalytic postcode of choice for those in the north – to rival NW3 in London for analysts clustered around Freud's house in Maresfield Gardens. Ruth had responded to a first trawl letter John Churcher and I sent out for people who might be willing to contribute to teaching on a psychoanalytic master's degree course in the city. She had an academic background in medical anthropology, and was keen to be on board for the course. Better still, she worked as a psychoanalytic psychotherapist and so, on the rebound from Frank Margison, I made an appointment to discuss therapy.

The meeting was in her apartment at the end of a leafy side road, a modern apartment block that housed a cosy, carpeted and rug-bestrewn space with armchairs and couches and oriental knick-knacks. Ruth, a grey-haired, bespectacled Jewish woman in her early seventies, with a strong Central European accent, invited me to sit down and asked if I would like a cup of tea. The accent was surely, I thought, Viennese, and I was torn between the sense that this was exactly the analyst for me, the real thing from Freud's own land, one of his people, and a suspicion that surely my psychoanalyst should not settle me down in her sitting room for tea and biscuits. They were plain digestive biscuits, and, more than that, they were offered to me with the story that the biscuit barrel that contained them had been a gift from Anna Freud. I was impressed, but also a little worried that this was rather too comfortable an encounter so far. She told me that her sister, Isca Salzberger-Wittenberg, was a Kleinian psychotherapist at the Tavistock Clinic.

"Well," I coughed nervously, "well, I am looking for a psychoanalyst." And, beginning to gabble, "I'm interested in the connection between psychoanalysis and politics, started being very interested in the work of Wilhelm Reich and then Erich Fromm." Ruth made a little face at the mention of Reich, but stopped me when I got to Fromm. "Erich Fromm," she said, "yes, I knew him very well." Good, I was encouraged, even if it was not the response I had anticipated. I said that I wanted to know more about psychoanalysis, what the process of psychoanalytic treatment was like as a personal experience, that I was a Marxist, and that the reason I liked Reich and Fromm so much was that they did attempt to connect the two domains.

Ruth told me that Fromm played the guitar very well. I sat on the edge of the couch balancing the teacup on the saucer and refused the offer of another biscuit. I ploughed on, saying that it was also important to me that I be able to question what psychoanalysis was as a historically-specific form of knowledge. Now she looked worried. "Do you have supervision?" I asked. She asked what I meant, and I described the process at Gaskell House. "Do you think I need supervision?" she asked, and, before I had a chance to reply – I was hesitating, not sure what the right answer to this was – she said she would certainly think about whether she should have supervision.

She said that perhaps we should now take time to reflect on our conversation after our meeting and that she would soon be in contact with me about it. I left feeling as I would leaving an elderly relative, not so much because of the tangle of miscommunication that characterises so much family interaction, in my family at any rate, but because I had had a conversation that was so very different from the one I expected. A week later Ruth phoned and dropped me. "I think it would be better," she said, "that we remain friends." This was as curious a formulation as those that comprised the meeting itself. I was rattled by this. I wondered if I had tried to set the terms of a possible analysis too high when I warned her that I wanted also to question psychoanalysis itself, that in this shopping expedition I had been too choosy, a difficult customer, one to avoid.

This had been but one meeting, so I wasn't sure what she meant about us being friends. I couldn't imagine speaking to her about myself, felt anxious at the thought of it, and imagined, instead, humouring her about what all her own personal links to psychotherapists meant to her. Perhaps it would have been a disaster. I told friends about what had happened, and heard from one former patient of Ruth's that they had been asked to do some shopping for her on occasion and had even been invited to tea one day with her other patients. My disappointment turned to relief at another fortunate escape – a rather symptomatic response – which then left me rather anxious about what therapy involved; turning disappointment into relief, into a sense that I was lucky to be free rather than face what it was I might have lost, was a defence of some kind, but as with every defence, one with consequences, costs. Where are they when you want them, these psychotherapists?

It was possible that I was being too cautious. I was certainly too cautious to go to my doctor and ask for a referral. This, not only because I was clearly one of the worried well, could have been put in a queue of lower-grade hypochondriacs who clearly did not need treatment but were clogging up the NHS, getting in the way of those who really did need help. This, more importantly, because asking for help in that way could be a route to a medical treatment in which the pathway and the endpoint would be out of my control. What demand could I possibly make for therapy on the NHS that would be serious enough to arrive at a psychotherapist I could trust, perhaps someone like me, working as an honorary therapist with little or no training in a place like Gaskell House, but not so serious that I would end up on medication as the cheaper and more obvious kind of treatment. I liked some of those who spoke at the Gaskell House meetings, but many of them were psychiatrists, and some of them, I thought, were too flaky to trust. This was a disturbing thought. I distrusted my own suspicious response, wondering who I *could* ask, if I was so quick to rule out my own colleagues as intimate interlocutors.

The local radical mental health groups, such as Mind, formerly the National Association for Mental Health, and Asylum Magazine radical mental health activists in Manchester, who were now busy setting up Hearing Voices groups, desperately wanted access to therapeutic services as an alternative to the drug pushers in the National Schizophrenia Fellowship. There were the counselling services at the Polytechnic that we invited speakers from. They were nice people, but dedicated to helping out with specific issues: Samaritans for those who were suicidal – no, that was not something I would want to admit to anyone else, even in therapy – Cruse for those who were bereaved, and so on. I hadn't even gone to Frank or Ruth with symptoms. The Frankfurt School theorist Max Horkheimer was turned away from analysis when he first asked because there was no symptom, only curiosity about the process, but the analyst took him on later when Max remembered that he sometimes felt anxious lecturing. There were no small-ads in the local press. There were listings of a few in the local Yellow Pages directory of businesses and services, but then how could I be sure that I wouldn't end up with someone even more off the wall than Ruth.

Don

I asked around for recommendations, and was given names that were always tentatively prefaced with the story that so-and-so was reputedly very good but you could never be sure, that so-and-so had been seen by a friend of a friend and they had seemed reliable. Some suggestions were balanced out with warnings, and sometimes the names were coupled with an anecdote about how they had been helpful to one friend but had been much disliked by another. Every first-hand account was charged with emotion, about therapists who had clearly listened and those who had clearly been uninterested, of those who had helped and those who had let their patients down.

One name recurred in the lists of those who were judged fine, as good enough: Don Feasey out in East Didsbury. He was on the edge, not centrally involved in any of the circles I moved in. I had never met him, and I decided this was very positive, for it meant that I was unlikely to encounter him elsewhere during the time I was in therapy with him. And those circles were good ones. He was linked in some way to the psychodrama scene, Jan and Stuart had mentioned him, somewhere on the outer edges of the NWIDP, his name was one recommended by acquaintances at Gaskell House, and he wrote for a small radical magazine called *Changes*, radical enough as well as good enough perhaps, and a writer, perhaps an academic, a sometime don. I gave him a go.

It wasn't that long after my other failed appointments, a matter of weeks, but I had devoted some time to this task of finding a therapist. We met first on a Friday afternoon in February 1993. He didn't offer me a cup of tea, but I liked him anyway, a greying, softly-spoken man in his sixties, I thought, perhaps Irish, perhaps not, I was piecing together an image of him from his name and his demeanour, and the kind of clothes that put him the broad category of what we, Erica and me, called 'cuddly jumper therapists', a very broad category that included Frank Margison – when he wasn't wearing a suit.

Don's house was a large cuddly-jumper kind of house, with a large bay window at the front, and a strong, wooden front door up a couple of steps. In you would go, over brown carpet, past cream walls, around to the left into the front room where there was a couch in the bay. He sat in a chair in front of one of the bookshelves, around to the left just into the room, and I sat opposite him, the couch to my right. A searching thoughtful look made me sense that he was giving his full attention to me when I spoke, when he asked me to sit down and to tell me why I was there. This time I just said I wanted to be in psychoanalytic psychotherapy. Silence. Looking. Thinking.

I said I was frightened and distrustful of psychiatrists and felt I needed to be in therapy if I was to be seeing a patient at Gaskell House. I didn't know what would be spoken of in those sessions there that would possibly stir up things for me, and I needed a place to reflect on who I was and how I might be affected. Out of the corner of my eye I could see a photo in the bookshelf of Sigmund Freud and his daughter Anna. Perhaps Don was an Anna Freudian. He was, I was sure. I asked when we would start. He said, "Well, I think we have." I think, though I cannot remember for sure, that he told me that I should pay £15 for a session, and that if I did not give more than 48 hours' notice, I should pay for missed sessions. In the second or third session I made a comment about the couch, and he said I should see how it felt there. I took off my shoes, and there I was.

I was with Don for nearly two years. Some early mornings I would be invited in, untie my bootlaces and lie on the couch waiting for him while he finished his breakfast – I think that's what he was doing, toast and marmalade smells sometimes wafted through from the back of the house.

These sessions were quite early in the morning. I would cycle over from Chorlton and then cycle afterwards up to campus to teach. Don seemed to like that I cycled, commenting one time that it was good to put a bit of effort in to coming along to therapy. "It shouldn't be too easy," he said. One thing that annoyed me was when he moralised, came out with little homilies, which sometimes extended to anecdotes. But I could cope with this, and perhaps this is something I learned to do in these sessions. That is, those donnish interventions were so softly done that I didn't feel them as intrusive, but let them wash over me, at times irritating as wasting time in the session I was paying for, and at times relieving as a bit of time for me to think without speaking, distancing rather than intruding.

I spoke of a time when I was with two schoolfriends in the wooded, sprawling grounds of Sundridge Park Management Centre, a place where my mother worked for a while as a secretary. I described us finding a tunnel down to the edge of a round, brick pit, sunk deep into the ground, about twenty feet down and twenty feet in circumference. We clambered down a rickety pile of planks and makeshift ladders, barely able to see, weak light filtered down through another small hole in the ground directly above us, and, as we made our way down, we destroyed the decaying means of entry and exit, so for a while we were trapped. One of us clambered out with our help, pushing his feet up and holding them steady on the debris piled up against the brick wall. He knelt at the top and encouraged us to follow him out, but now the task for us was more difficult. Now we were two, with not enough light to see what there was around the rest of the pit and not enough strength for one of us to climb up and the other to stretch up to push up the other. The longer we waited, the lower the light, the more we exerted ourselves the more tired we became. I said I sometimes dreamed of this. Here I am in this pit, I said, but I don't know how to get out. Don eventually said he was surprised that I did not imagine a magical solution to the problem I was trapping myself in; I could have imagined that another tunnel might have opened up in the wall leading to somewhere else entirely. What did he mean by saying this?

I spotted another photo of Anna Freud in the bookshelf one day, or perhaps it was the same one, and this renewed my search for evidence that Don was an Anna Freudian. Her 1936 book *The Ego and the Mechanisms of Defence* was a classic text that I referred to in my teaching, for it summarised and extended her father's own scattered references to defences like 'rationalisation' and 'intellectualisation', the ways we are able to neatly explain away slips of the tongue and dreams, or use psychoanalytic terminology to describe them without really connecting with what is going on. Rationalisation was the work of everyday common-sense resistance to psychoanalysis: the busy work of the rational ego that thinks of itself as the core of the self, and puts down any intrusions or unexpected events to chance or devises convenient explanations that everyone else will also be happy to agree on. Intellectualisation is the mainstay of academic psychoanalysis, and satisfying to the ego too; references to trauma and desire are safely enclosed in a rationalist shell of hermetic explanation that all the more effectively keeps the unconscious at bay. We can speak about things in such a way as to keep them separate from us; our language, even in the clinic, can then function as a wall, protecting us, ego speech.

Finding a photo, fixing on it, thinking about why Don was saying certain things to me in terms of the intellectual frame that I supposed was guiding him, was just such a protective device, a defence mechanism. Anna Freud spelled out the many different ways we protect ourselves, which include projection and denial, and defence mechanisms became the leitmotif of her version of ego-psychology, complementing the categorisation of different kinds of defence mechanisms by George Vaillant, in the US, who sorted them into psychotic, immature, neurotic and mature kinds, this last including altruism and humour. Far from breaking down or breaking through the defence mechanisms in therapy, then, the task is rather to reconfigure them; reinforcing those defences that are helpful and questioning the value of those that are destructive and self-sabotaging. Perhaps this is what the suggestion that I might find imaginative solutions to my imagined incarceration in the brick pit meant. Perhaps Don was accentuating one kind of defence mechanism while questioning another.

It was very difficult to spot what Don was doing as being specifically Anna Freudian. In the second year he was ill, and we didn't meet for about six weeks, and then, when we resumed the sessions, he commented that I hadn't asked him how he was. Perhaps he was guiding me towards employing a more 'mature' defence mechanism, showing some altruistic concern for how he was feeling. As far as I was concerned, the therapy was already riddled enough with transference, ranging from my image of him as being a rather grandfatherly figure to the picture I had of him standing waiting for me to pay him, slightly stooping, taking the money, more, I thought at the time, like an itinerant gardener, his jumper then looking not so comfy, a little more worn. I oscillated between feelings of tenderness and contempt, one emotional response no doubt functioning in relation to the other along dimensions of schizoid fantasy, bad, psychotic, or suppression, mature, good.

Sometimes Don chuckled at what I said, sometimes at his own anecdotes; his favourites were about a novelist, who was apparently an acquaintance, who seemed to function in the session as a model of how not to behave. Perhaps he was modelling what it was to be a good person, and this would be very much in line with some assumptions in ego-psychology, that the ideal end of analysis is when the ego of the patient identifies with, and models itself on the ego of the analyst. This would need to be an analyst who has already, we suppose, been cleansed of bad inclinations and who has learned to use mature defence mechanisms against unhealthy ideas.

There were some things Don said that I would not have said to my patient at Gaskell House. I imagined Jean (Rawsthorne) would have sharply warned me against anecdotes about who I knew and what I thought about academics and politics. I couldn't easily filter out elements of the different sessions and map them onto different models. Perhaps my attempt to do so was a dead end. My time with my patient Martin came to an end and shortly after that I finished with Don. In the last session he said I had done quite well, perhaps gone as far as I was able in the time we were together. I didn't like this. I should have done better, and his comment might have meant that I was unable to. There was a silence. "This is like waiting at a station for a train to leave isn't it," he said. It was very apposite, for I am someone who does not like to wait around at a station waiting for friends to go, or for them to hang around when I am leaving. I like to get it over and done with quickly, in haste. I agreed with Don, had to linger a little longer, and eventually it was time to go.

This looked like therapy, this third close encounter with psychoanalysis. It was, but it was also research. It was research into psychoanalysis. Then it was how to teach about psychoanalytic research that was to draw me even closer to psychoanalysis and, after some respite during these few years in the company of the British tradition, back to Lacan.

8

RESEARCH

Studying and experiencing

I should already have known. It had been problematic enough teaching about psychoanalysis within the frame of the university as a form of psychotherapy, and now it was to be just as problematic teaching about psychoanalysis as a form of research. The academic context demands an objective appraisal of knowledge that is quite impossible, and I discovered that many psychoanalysts are so attached to their favourite form of knowledge that a subjective engagement with the topic is also hedged around with dangers. The process of constructing a psychoanalytic studies degree course did, however, at least give me access to some debates about what it would mean to 'return to Freud' and, along the way, to debates about the nature of 'trauma' in Freudian theory.

Click

A new discipline, psychoanalytic studies, appeared at the University of Kent at Canterbury in the form of a master's programme in 1985, and the Centre for Psychoanalytic Studies was founded there a year later. The MA at Kent was a magnet for a new wave of students from a range of existing academic disciplines, including some who had worked with us in the Discourse Unit, our research group at the Poly in Manchester. Genie Georgaca, who had spent time as an Erasmus Exchange student from Greece at the University of Manchester, went to Kent to take that psychoanalytic studies course before returning to Manchester for her PhD with us. Dan Heggs, who had been a psychology undergraduate student with us at the Poly, was enthused enough by the 'Psychoanalysis and society' final-year option to take that path too. Students at Kent, including Luke Thurston and Heather Menzies, were in first cohorts. I stayed with Heather when I went to Kent to give my 'Melanie Klein and Alien Abduction' paper to the student group there.

The driving force behind the MA was Martin Stanton, who styled himself as a Laplanchian, a follower of the French psychoanalyst Jean Laplanche. Laplanche would have been best known to academics as the co-author, with Jean-Bertrand Pontalis, of the invaluable encyclopaedic dictionary translated into English in 1973 as *The Language of Psychoanalysis*. Laplanche was once a Trotskyist in France, and, after working in the French Resistance during the Second World War, was a founding member in 1948 of the far-left group Socialisme ou Barbarie. Such a political trajectory was not that unusual in psychoanalytic circles.

Many of Freud's associates had been members or sympathisers of communist parties in Central Europe, and the leader of the Anna Freudians in London, Joseph Sandler, had once been a member of the Trotskyist Fourth International in South Africa. Laplanche, who had made the choice of psychoanalysis over politics after leaving Socialisme ou Barbarie, was closely associated with Jacques Lacan during the time of the first rifts with the IPA in 1953, eventually opting to move over to the official IPA franchise organisation in Paris in 1963. He was rehabilitated sufficiently to be able to speak at the Institute of Psychoanalysis in London in June 1984, which is where I first encountered him.

Laplanche told a joke at the beginning of that lecture, about a man who thought he was a seed, who was frantically frightened of the chickens in the yard chasing after him, he thought, and ready to eat him up. He was frightened enough at this paranoid thought that the chickens would eat him because he was a seed that he went to a psychoanalyst, and after a long period of intensive work on this delusion that he was a seed, was cured. He no longer thought he was a seed. His psychoanalyst was passing by the man's farm a while later and saw his patient running scared from the chickens. "What's up," the analyst said, "you are not a seed." The man replied, "You know that, I know that, but do the chickens know that?"

This is one opening to a key question in psychoanalysis concerning the importance of not so much identity and the set of personal beliefs one has about oneself but of the way we live our identity in relation to others, of what we attribute to others, what we imagine others want of us. We live in relation to a diffuse, generalised sense of otherness, Jacques Lacan had argued, to a 'big Other' in whose shadow, and for whom, we live so much of our lives. In its most paranoiac aspect there is the idea that there is something or somebody else who is behind the scenes pulling the strings of the big Other as society or cultural institutions; and Lacan was to shift during the course of his career from a warning that there is no Other of the Other to a more fundamental assertion that, when it comes down to it, and as a lesson of psychoanalysis, the Other does not exist.

Laplanche's own particular innovative take on this question of the relationship between the nascent self and others came in the shape of an approach to trauma that he conceptualised in terms of 'enigmatic signifiers', which are fragments of indecipherable speech or action, sound or image, that function as a message to the infant. While Freud is often falsely accused of failing to take child sexual abuse seriously, because he shifted attention to sexual fantasies on the part of the infant, Laplanche deepened the psychoanalytic accounts of how those sexual fantasies become organised around the actions of the parents or significant others. The infant's carers are, of course, sexual beings, and their interaction with the infant will include much that is inexplicable. Child sexual abuse has always been taken seriously by psychoanalysis, but Laplanche's understanding of the way that the implicit abuse, hidden in messages that the infant is confused by and unable to process at a time when it is helpless, also has consequences for every real and fantasised form of traumatic childhood event.

Enigmatic signifiers stick in the memory as undigested remnants of childhood, and the way they are activated and flooded with meaning is central to a psychoanalytic account of development, an account of the relationship between adulthood and childhood that is radically anti-developmental. This relationship hinges around time, and a concept that Laplanche and Pontalis in their dictionary of psychoanalysis praise Lacan for retrieving, after the event, from Freud. In Freud, Laplanche and Pontalis point out, we find the notion of *Nachträglichkeit*, or, to Anglo-neologise it, 'afterwardsness'. Psychoanalytic time is not linear, not ordered in terms of cause and effect, which is something that psychologists and psychiatrists, who are wedded to simple causal models of development, find difficult to understand. Things are given meaning after the event, crucially so in the case of trauma, so that early events that are disturbing, nonsensical, uncomfortable, are given meaning by a later event. It is this chiming of a later event, perhaps an unpleasant sexual encounter, with an earlier sexual event that turns the earlier event into something that is traumatic. This can be summed up in the Laplanchean dictum: 'it takes two traumas to make a trauma.'

Perhaps the chicken man's analysis did not go far enough. At any rate, the problem revolves around the relationship with what the chicken wants, what is supposed of the chicken as Other to the man. Psychoanalysts would suspect that there is something that happened earlier that is being activated as an unconscious trauma, something to do with chickens, who knows, and this is then driving the poor man mad as he projects his paranoiac fears onto the chickens in his yard.

The implicitly Laplanchean frame for the MA 'Psychoanalytic studies' at Kent was useful as a way of linking a number of different psychoanalytic traditions, enabling students to work on Lacan or Klein or on other psychoanalytic traditions. It was from Genie Georgaca's coursework at Kent, for example, that I was first introduced to an amazing 1989 book called *The Sublime Object of Ideology*, in which the author, Slovenian Slavoj Žižek, claimed that Marx invented the psychoanalytic symptom and that Lacan knew this. We spent a holiday in Greece with Genie, where I read Žižek's book as well as *Counter-Clock World* by Philip K. Dick, a science fiction novel in which time operates in a most weird, quasi-psychoanalytic way, in reverse.

Psychoanalytic studies as an academic programme is, of course, structured around a number of paradoxes, one of which revolves around the relationship between understanding and time. If Laplanche and Lacan and their readings of Freud on *Nachträglichkeit* were right, then our experience of the world and the sense we make of it is always in some way 'retroactive'. The 'working through' that psychoanalytic practitioners speak of is not so much a direct appreciation and sedimentation in consciousness of what has been discovered in therapy, but a strange looping of reflection in which what has been said and heard in the sessions is continually reconfigured. What seemed insignificant or puzzling at one moment is thrown into relief, becomes active as an idea, either consciously or unconsciously, at some later point. In my sessions with Martin at Gaskell House, for example, I would faithfully relay to him from my supervision an interpretation of what he was talking about, to find that he made a quite different sense of that interpretation to the one intended, sometimes ignoring it altogether and then, surprisingly and unpredictably, referring or alluding to it in a later session.

Now we were faced with a number of problems, tangles that we three, Frank Margison, John Churcher and me, tussled over. Our psychoanalytic programme would be composed of discrete modules, we thought, which would make the composition of the degree programme containable and also make it possible to stitch together contributions from the three component institutions. No one aspect of psychoanalysis is really separable from the others, however, and, more importantly, there is no real agreement as to which aspects are foundational and which are supplementary. Even more contentious was the related question as to which components are necessary and which 'optional'.

Frank was interested, of course, in the clinical relevance of the theoretical work, theoretical work that, he did agree, could be put in a first module called 'Freudian foundations'. We could agree that Freud was at the heart of the programme even if we found it difficult to agree which bits of Freud should be included there. Frank was willing to defer to the theory at this point, and it was an academically sound programme that attracted him and would, he thought, attract psychotherapists. They might even gain grounding in the theory that they had not really had in their own practically-focused trainings.

But then, 'modules' should surely be linked together in a sequence, in what modular programmes referred to as 'progression', something that effectively unravelled much of the modular framework. There was an 'Applied psychology' modular programme, for example, that had been relocated from Salford University to the University of Manchester, and that the Polytechnic contributed to. A group of us at the Poly ran the qualitative methods course, and we knew from that experience how difficult it was both to reflect critically, qualitatively on the standard psychology that most students already knew about and, at the same time, to provide something that was more foundational for students who hadn't yet been exposed to some of the more mechanistic experimental approaches.

Nevertheless, we could make it work well enough because there were competing views about what counted in psychology across the whole degree programme. A level playing field made it possible for qualitative and critical approaches to find a voice. In the case of this psychoanalytic studies programme, where we wanted to agree on a coherent approach that would give students a good grounding in psychoanalytic theory and practice, and take responsibility for that as a course team, things were more complicated. We were still trapped in a linear course structure that relied on the assumption that students accumulate knowledge and develop their expertise.

Develop

John Churcher had an interesting relationship with time. Don't we all. Meetings with Frank about the possibility of setting up our own psychoanalytic studies master's programme at Manchester would be strictly governed by the clock, well, by John's watch, which he would consult as he arrived and when he advised us that he would have a taxi ready outside. He had calculated that the time and money spent on taxis would be more efficient than driving a car, quite possibly true, and had a packed schedule into which psychoanalytic studies would be slotted. His training at the Institute of Psychoanalysis was exactly that, a gruelling sequence of train journeys and evening meetings, which meant that he often had to travel down and stay in London overnight. He had to fit in his own personal analysis five times a week, and seminars, and supervision for the clinical cases he undertook. I was impressed, and thought it was a bit crazy. The psychoanalytic studies programme was another bit of the jigsaw, an opportunity for relaying psychoanalysis to students and, if at all possible, to psychotherapists. That created a particular tension in our discussions, in the way we conceptualised the relationship between academic research and clinical practice.

For John Churcher, the clinical practice was the baseline for what he called the 'experience' of psychoanalysis, and beneath this was a more fundamental assumption about the nature of psychoanalysis itself: that it was fundamentally true, and that 'experience' of the world as psychoanalysis described it made clinical work necessary and possible. I was engaged with psychoanalysis, but I was not a convert, and I did not want to evangelise about it. By now, however, I was absorbed in psychoanalysis and John's intense engagement with it was something to marvel at. He would remind me, for example, how implausible was Jeffrey Masson's claim in his 1984 book *Assault on Truth*, that Freud had abandoned his 'seduction theory' because he wanted to curry favour with the psychiatric establishment, because he wanted to fit in. Freud's first approach to trauma, in which child sexual abuse was treated as the cause of hysterical distress, was shocking, but that seduction theory was not at all replaced with a more socially-convenient explanation. It was, if anything, more shocking when Freud then claimed that every one of us is beset by fantasies of abuse that at some point are rendered traumatic to us. It simply was not true that Freud and later psychoanalysts did not take child sexual abuse seriously – there are references to it in many of the case histories – and the turn to fantasy and the development of psychoanalysis was bound up with a shift from saying one thing that would be unpopular to something completely outrageous, subversive. It was then that he became really quite isolated. I learned over and over again from John during our discussions that psychoanalysis needed to be taken seriously, but that, I thought, was because the cultural conditions that gave rise to it *make* it something serious to us.

The idea that psychoanalysis and psychoanalytic description were, culturally, historically specific was anathema to John. He had a good understanding of Marxism, and was a radical force in groups like European Nuclear Disarmament

(END), an alternative, more moderate group, a slightly more muted version of the Campaign for Nuclear Disarmament, one that was being promoted by 'Euro-communist' and social democratic activists. However, just as END adopted a more cautious approach and distanced itself from the far left in the peace movement, so John was very suspicious of attempts to link psychoanalysis and Marxism. "Just remember," he said on several occasions, as he gave me a meaningful, warning look over his moustache, "what happened to Wilhelm Reich." The implication, I guess, was that if I carried on down that ultra-left path, I'd eventually go mad. It was a friendly warning, but he meant it. Our conceptual differences over psychoanalysis were always tangled up with political differences.

The placeholder for Reich as a radical force in psychoanalysis in Manchester in the 1980s was Lacan. Or, rather, the signifier 'Lacan' evoked a possible connection with a radical rereading of Freud, much more so than did 'Reich'. This was, perhaps, because Reich conjured up a vision of an already-existing, energetic unconscious comprising libidinal forces that sought release – the pressure-cooker hydraulic model of the mind – while Lacan was more in tune with the 'social constructionist' idea that what was repressed was created in the very process of repression. In addition, Lacan was gaining in popularity in some academic circles even though the theoretical framework presented itself as at the margins. The difficulty of his writing, his inaccessibility, was a win-win; he was an intellectual force *and* not everyone understood what he was saying.

This representation of Lacan held a double danger for me in the context of our course development discussions. First, because I was not convinced that Lacan himself was really that radical. Lacanian theory had entered Britain in the 1970s through debates around ideology and sexuality, promoted by academics who were attracted to the French Marxist philosopher Louis Althusser and by feminists who saw the turn to language and culture in Lacan's work and the work of some of his followers as being more open to links between subjectivity and social change. Althusser was a structuralist who argued that ideology and the unconscious were 'eternal', and so I was doubtful that his contribution was really so helpful as a link between revolutionary change in society and personal change. There had been a sea change in feminist debates, for example after the publication of Juliet Mitchell's wonderful 1974 book *Psychoanalysis and Feminism*, which reviewed the sexual liberation motifs in Reich as well as Lacanian ideas. Žižek was also beginning to reactivate the link between psychoanalysis and Marxism. The image of Lacanian theory as radical, and my misgivings about this, made the signifier 'Lacan' an uncomfortable one to be associated with in discussions about 'Psychoanalytic studies'.

The second reason Lacan was dangerous in this context, and someone I had misgivings about, was because these ideas came to Britain mainly through academic culture and literary and film theory, and this made it seem as if Lacan was a countercultural or political writer disconnected from clinical practice. I didn't want to embrace Lacan or the signifier 'Lacan' because that would tie me to a framework I was not completely happy with, and, worse, in this context it would tie me to someone who didn't seem to contribute to debates over the practice of psychoanalysis. I was still ambivalent about clinical psychoanalysis, but we needed to take it seriously as a domain in which psychoanalysis was put to work. Over-attachment, over-identification with Lacan might jeopardise that.

John and Frank were sympathetic enough to Lacan to want to give his reading of Freud space on the course, but Lacan was arguing for more than merely a new reading in his own school of psychoanalysis that was founded in Paris in 1964 and that then sprouted affiliates around the world in the years since. Lacan argued that his account was itself the strictest most loyal heritage of the founders of psychoanalysis. He asserted at one point, for example, that just as Marx had distanced himself from followers who claimed they were Marxist, that he, Lacan, was not 'Lacanian' but Freudian. Lacan claimed to 'return to Freud', and that the IPA tradition had effectively betrayed its supposed master. The stakes were high, with an apparently neutral historical exegesis of Freudian texts in the first 'Freudian foundations' module, which we did agree would have to be first, being pitted against a version of the module that already embedded Lacanian concepts. Here was an emphasis on language in the development of psychoanalysis as a 'talking cure' that enabled Freud to shift from a physiological to a psychical notion of distress and treatment, and to the notion of *Nachträglichkeit*, which embedded in the practice an authentically psychoanalytic notion of trauma and time.

The first time I met John he used a phrase that indicated a point of connection between Lacan and Klein, and when he repeated it several times over the following years it became a signifier of the journey he was taking from Lacanian to full-blown, hard-line Kleinian psychoanalysis. The phrase was '*corps morcelé*', something I had to look up after our first meeting and after I had disentangled it from what I heard as 'cormorsellay'. *Corps morcelé* is the body in pieces, hallucinatory images and sensations of the fragmented biological being that the infant is subjected to during its trajectory through the mirror-stage. The illusory unity of self, of the foundations of the ego modelled on the image of the other in the mirror-stage, unleashes fantasies of what lies outside that self-sufficient, jubilant self-identity of the infant, horrific Bosch-like images of what would happen if that identity disintegrated. Lacan had been most impressed with Klein's 1932 book *The Psycho-Analysis of Children*, offering to translate it into French when he met her at the Sixteenth IPA Congress in Zurich in 1949, but then lost the manuscript before he had done so. What he saw there was a description of paranoiac phantasies of the body in pieces, good and bad objects, which were very close to what he had already conceptualised as the nightmarish unconscious mirror-world of the infant, anxious to buttress its own sense of self.

Klein argued that the infant is envious of what others have, and there is a desire to take it and spoil it. The paranoid-schizoid position she describes is infused with envious, spoiling spite directed at the first good object, the breast, and attempts to enter it and destroy it. This paranoid-schizoid position eventually gives way to the depressive position in which there is a sense of gratitude for what is offered, a sense of goodness in others and the self. The shift from paranoid-schizoid position to depressive position is thus correlated with a shift from envy to gratitude. However, these positions are not, strictly speaking, developmental stages, and we are beset as adults by paranoid-schizoid phantasies that are addressed in analysis, in the transference as the analysand enviously attacks and attempts to enter and spoil the inside of the analyst, with the end of analysis marked by gratitude and attainment of the depressive position.

Even though this was not really a developmental stage, any more than Lacan's mirror-stage was, it could be interpreted as such, and so child observation became one of the signature aspects of psychoanalytic training in the Institute of Psychoanalysis. The Anna Freudians worked with children and observed children, attended to the attachment bonds that were forged between infant and mother. The object-relations independent Middle Group psychoanalysts around Winnicott observed the capacity for containment by the mother and the attachment of the infant to transitional objects that lay at the boundaries between inside and outside the self. And the Kleinians observed infantile shifts between envy and gratitude.

Mrs Klein was respectfully asked one day how it was possible to really observe whether the infant was envious or not. She replied, while pointing at an infant in its mother's arms, "Now it is envious," pause, "and now it is not." This is something that Kleinian psychoanalysts in training would be expected to see for themselves, and to use as evidence for the knowledge base they used in the clinic with adults, their patients.

John insisted that there should be some space in the psychoanalytic studies programme for infant observation, as it would give students an experience of psychoanalysis. I was wary about this. It seemed to wipe away the 'afterwardsness' of psychoanalysis, and to insist on one correct interpretation of child behaviour, as if we could see into the minds of infants. It seemed that we would be trapped in a version of psychoanalysis that was linear and developmental, and, worse, would be turning it into a world view, as if psychoanalysis was indubitably true everywhere and as if we should teach it as evangelists who wanted our students to believe it was true too.

Sympathetic though they were to Lacan, neither John nor Frank wanted to allow that theory to operate as the cuckoo in the nest. John's training at the IPA was drawing him closer to a Kleinian framework, and so he quite understandably wanted that to be fully represented in the course. I agreed that it should be there, and saw our course as being located quite explicitly in the 'British tradition', one that included Klein and Winnicott and the whole gamut of object-relations theories. We were able to hold things together from time to time in our course development discussions by deflecting attention onto our shared enemies. We drew the boundaries of the programme around a version of 'psychoanalysis' that kept Jung out. Frank could live with that, and we didn't tell his mentor, Bob Hobson, who had, anyway, left the SAP (the Jungian Society of Analytical Psychologists) a while ago.

Print

We were shadowed by two institutional conflicts around and beyond us that we could not evade so easily. Our big Others. They intersected. One was the relationship between the IPA in London and other rival training organisations. The IPA line was that only those who had been trained at its Institute of Psychoanalysis could be called ‘psychoanalysts’; anyone else training in another institution in Britain was a pretender to the title. There was an uneasy truce with the Jungians, who agreed not to claim the title psychoanalyst and stayed, instead, with the ‘analytical psychology’ label that Jung himself had adopted when he broke with Freud in 1913. This institutional line would mean that Genie Georgaca, who returned from the Kent psychoanalytic studies programme in 1993 for her PhD on psychotic language, under my supervision, should not be recognised as a psychoanalyst when she completed the parallel training she was taking at CFAR, the Centre for Freudian Analysis and Research, a Lacanian training organisation in London. John knew Genie well from her time as an Erasmus student at the University of Manchester, but his own allegiance to the IPA was strong, and he defended that organisation’s line on rival groups: they were not psychoanalysts.

The other institutional conflict was between rival academic institutions where the power play between them was just as insidious and corrosive as the one between the IPA and the Lacanians. This conflict brought into play the question of class alongside the question of status. Unlike the Jungians, who were accorded grudging respect as a separate strand, the Lacanians were viewed as a threat, and looked down upon as upstarts, arrivistes on the British scene, less than psychoanalysts, perhaps as idiosyncratic psychoanalytic psychotherapists, but nothing more, maybe worse. CFAR had been founded as recently as 1985 as the only Lacanian clinical training programme in Britain. It charged much less for its training, but that training was also viewed by the IPA as less rigorous. While the roll call of members of the British Psychoanalytical Society boasted double-barrelled names and included members of the House of Lords, and many members of the Society of Analytical Psychologists were similarly well-heeled, CFAR members were treated as if they were, at best, nouveau riche, little better than the lowest of the low, the middle-class and even working-class counsellors.

This pyramid hierarchy mapped onto the shape of academic provision in class-sensitive Britain, with respect-contempt relationships between psychoanalysts, psychotherapists and counsellors replicated in the relationships between the original, ancient, most prestigious universities like Oxford and Cambridge, the Red Bricks founded in the wake of nineteenth-century industrialisation in cities like Manchester, and the 1960s ‘plate glass’ institutions that included places like the University of Kent at Canterbury. John was sensitive to this hierarchy, commenting when I first met him that his own Red Brick university in Manchester was ‘provincial’, rated less than Oxbridge. My place, along with the rest of the polytechnics, was granted university charter status in 1992, and complemented the other university in the city in terms of class intake. The two institutions’ rivalry made joint work between academics very difficult; the old Polytechnic, now MMU, Manchester Metropolitan University, was proudly continuing the legacy of local government bureaucratic surveillance of every course development, something that it pitted against the more lax, less formal approach of the older, more patrician university up the road.

I admit it, I was impatient to get the degree programme running, and exasperated by the delays. Our two institutions would not agree to a 'joint programme', and so the sensible default option was a course based at the University of Manchester and linked to Gaskell House, which was already institutionally located in the same fold as part of the university hospital, with MMU as a partner, a junior partner. I applied for a job in the psychology department at the University of Manchester, but was not short-listed, and heard from an inside source that the head of department had said he would only have me there over his dead body. There was no way that they would allow what I wrote about in a department that valued its scientific experimental status. John was already sidelined because of his interest in psychoanalysis, so it was a bit crazy to think that I could move in and use the place as a base for psychoanalytic studies.

I was enraged, yes, envious. Maybe Klein was right. I admit I behaved badly, sending out an announcement that the MA 'Psychoanalytic studies' at MMU would start in September 1996. We already had 'Freudian foundations' as a module on the books, Genie had taught it as a stand-alone course, and I reckoned we could go it alone. "What have you done?" John said when he found out. He never forgave me and I can't blame him. Our first and only intake at MMU was of three students. Erica ran the 'Freudian foundations' module as a reading group, left behind to take charge of the programme after I took up an academic post at another institution shortly afterwards, and so her interest in group analysis framed discussion of psychoanalysis for these three. Group analysis was not an approach we had factored into our map of psychoanalytic theories on the course, but now it opened up another dimension of psychoanalysis, and another route to training.

In another diversion, but another step closer to psychoanalysis, I was being drawn to the idea that I might myself train as an analyst. The process of working with Frank and John had impressed on me the importance of practical links between clinical work and political change. For all of our conceptual differences, we each saw psychoanalysis as a liberating personal and social project, and the wider discussions with other therapists also drove that home to me. Malign institutional divisions, which were relayed into our passion for psychoanalytic studies, made it impossible. I could feel myself being swept along by forces beyond my control. One thing was for sure, and it was not only because I was reading some great political analyses by psychoanalytic writers, my ambivalence to psychoanalysis had been transformed into another kind of ambivalence that now took as its coordinates psychoanalysis discourse as such. Perhaps you can sense the shift of emphasis between the first four chapters of this book and these last four in which I was engaging more deeply, whether I liked it or not, in psychoanalysis. Those around me were talking of training, and even when I resisted the idea I heard myself contemplating the possibility. In the beginning were the words. They touched something. That process of psychoanalytic training is what I turn to in the following four chapters.

9

TRAINING

In group analysis

Now I am in training, almost. In this chapter I puzzle over group analysis, an approach to therapy in the group by the group that operates with many different theoretical frameworks, not all of them psychoanalytic. I am asking myself whether this might provide the most thoroughly social approach to personal experience and treatment. Group analysis draws attention to a more fundamental question, what it means to be 'social', with a theory of social and historical context that enables the approach to operate in tandem with many forms of psychoanalysis.

Large

Adele Mittwoch followed up her question about whether I ever cried – I had said yes – with this rather sharp interpretation: "You don't want to do this training at all do you." This is 1996. She didn't mean this as a question, and it was pretty useless for me to stumble and stutter that yes, of course I did, of course I wanted to train as a group analyst. Why? What is group analysis anyway?

Freud took a dim view of groups, and the key term in the title of his 1921 book *Group Psychology and the Analysis of the Ego* was, quite typically, mistranslated from the German *Massenpsychologie*, 'mass psychology', which he intended to refer to a much wider phenomenon than a restricted focus on 'groups' implied. The examples Freud chose to illustrate how a particular figure or idea comes to stand in place of the ego-ideal and bind together each ego of followers in a collective, as a form of identification, included the church, the army and parliamentary assemblies. These are large, well-organised institutions rather than the kinds of boiling rabble that other theorists of crowd psychology had already described and decried. Although Freud was rather suspicious of mass politics, one of the points he wanted to make in his group psychology book was that every apparently individual psychology is a form of social psychology, it always involves other people.

Psychoanalysis itself is, or should be, a thoroughly social analysis, conceptualising the formation of the individual ego as an assemblage of relationships with significant others. We patch together a particular version of the ego from those figures, and so we are who we have identified with in the past. This is also why transference in psychoanalytic treatment works, and why it is such a hazardous task for the psychoanalyst to guess which particular significant other is being brought to life again as an analysand relates to them in the clinic. It is never merely only one, and that is why psychoanalysts who interpret the transference in order to help bring the phenomenon into focus risk narrowing things down and misinterpreting what is going on.

Group analysts do most of their work in small groups, but are mindful of Freud's comments and the wider context, and are able to work with transference as it manifests itself in contradictory and complex forms in the clinic. The presence of seven or eight other people in a clinical group gives ample opportunity for transference to be established in such a way that many significant others can be made present, experienced in the here and now; relationships are reimagined, symbolised, and conflicts with those others worked through.

The approach was launched as a specific modality of psychoanalytic treatment in the UK during the Second World War, and institutionalised in the 1950s after the war by Siegmund Heinrich Fuchs, an émigré psychoanalyst who had fled the Nazis in 1933. He changed his name to S. H. Foulkes, and was usually referred to as Michael. Foulkes had attended Wilhelm Reich's seminars, and was appointed director of the clinic at the Frankfurt Psychoanalytic Institute, which was based in the same building as the Frankfurt Institute for Social Research, the Frankfurt School. Foulkes was one of the psychoanalysts who Ernest Jones, leader of the British Psychoanalytical Society, was able to get out of Germany in the 1930s. He arrived in Britain in 1933 with his wife and children, and then gained a British medical qualification so he could join the British Psychoanalytical Society, in which he became a training analyst in the 'B-Group', that is, with followers of Anna Freud. The psychoanalytic group psychotherapy sessions he conducted while in Exeter, in the south west of Britain, at the beginning of the war prepared him for a series of interventions at the Northfield Military Neurosis Centre. on the edge of Birmingham in the Midlands.

Northfield was the seedbed for two key strands of psychoanalytic group work in Britain, and relationships between the two have often been strained. Psychoanalysts drafted into the military had the task of dealing with battle-shocked soldiers – those who had been subjected to classical 'mass psychology' and trauma in their own units – and re-equipping them psychically for return to combat. The context in which the soldiers had suffered was also, crucially, a social context in which psychoanalysts were expected to revivify the sense of a common cause, team spirit in the body of the army, esprit de corps.

A first strand of group psychotherapy around the Kleinian psychoanalyst Wilfred Bion became embedded in the work of the Tavistock Institute and Tavistock Clinic, two influential institutions in the new National Health Service after the war, and so the followers of Bion had a power base from which to propagate their own understanding of what happened at Northfield and to advance their own version of appropriate therapeutic interventions. This version of Northfield was written up by Bion and another psychoanalyst, John Rickman, in the medical journal *The Lancet* in 1943. These interventions would be directed at the whole group, characterising the emotional atmosphere in a group as being 'angry', for example, and often relied on an understanding of different modes of defence enacted by a group.

Bion's description was of three 'basic assumption states' – of 'dependency' as the singling out of a saviour who will protect the group, of 'pairing' between two members that the rest of the group listen to in the belief they will produce something valuable, and 'fight-flight' in which the group is mobilised either to flee or to aggressively attack those viewed as threatening it. One can see how Bion's aims at Northfield, to highlight the purpose of the group of soldiers and encourage reflection on the system of relationships that hold it together, were part of the military agenda and linked with other work at the Tavistock on social systems by researchers like Elliott Jaques and Isabel Menzies Lyth noticing systems that could sometimes also be pathological.

Foulkes' own representation of what he called the 'Northfield Experiments', a second strand of group psychotherapy, one that does not mention either Bion or Rickman, builds on small-group work with the soldiers as part of what was effectively a 'therapeutic community'. The work with the men in the hospital was linked with broader community initiatives, liaising with employers in the area who might find work for the men, for example, something that became increasingly important after the war ended. Foulkes spent much longer at Northfield than Bion, who was there for only six weeks, and saw the group work as part of a much longer-term project, including how to adapt the men to civil society rather than simply get them ready to return to their units and fight again. After the war, a number of different group therapeutic models were tried out at Northfield, including Moreno's psychodrama.

Foulkes' own approach to group therapy, and to what became known as 'group analysis', was much more focused on the needs of individuals as members of a group than Bion's, avoiding 'whole group' interpretations, and having the analyst function as a 'conductor'. Foulkes argued that this kind of analysis was by the group and of the group, including the conductor. There was thus a subtle dialectic between what individuals brought to the group, particular preoccupations that were played out through the transference enacted in relation to members of the group, including the conductor, and what was created in the group. The to and fro and intersecting patterns of talk in the group constituted it as an analytic group, which Foulkes referred to as the 'matrix'. A Group Analytic Society was founded in London in 1952, and a training institute, the Institute of Group Analysis, in 1971. Foulkes died in a group of a heart attack in 1976. Old analysts who were present still talk about that.

Foulkes was the theorist behind group analysis, but there is another figure, often overlooked in the clinical discussions, who provides the closest to a social theory for group analysis, Norbert Elias. Elias was close to Foulkes during his time in Frankfurt, a figure working on the fringes of the Frankfurt School alongside Erich Fromm. After he fled Germany in 1933, he eventually ended up in Britain where he reconnected with his former supervisor, the sociologist Karl Mannheim, at the London School of Economics, where he worked as a research assistant. He finally got a teaching post at the University of Leicester in 1954, where he was influential on a new generation of academics interested in the sociology of sport. Sport is one aspect of what Elias called 'the civilizing process', which he described in detail in a 1939 book with that title, the first volume of which was published in English in 1969.

Michel Foucault acknowledged, in interviews conducted shortly before he died, that there were close similarities between his own account of the intimate link between surveillance and confession and those of the Frankfurt School, those to be found in classic texts such as Theodor Adorno and Max Horkheimer's *Dialectic of Enlightenment* first published in 1944. Norbert Elias's book on the civilizing process is also very close to Foucault's own genealogy, a historical analysis of everyday and institutional practices that traces how our experience of ourselves as separate individuals is bound up with institutional processes through which we become categorised and defined, regulated, and able to self-regulate, our behaviour alongside others. Elias's *The Civilizing Process* includes a detailed examination of the development of such taken-for-granted, everyday practices as using a handkerchief to blow our noses or cutlery to eat our food. One of Elias's last projects before he died in 1990 was to walk with his shoelaces undone in different countries and note when and how people pointed this out to him.

It is possible to interpret the psychoanalytic process as effectively enabling what Foucault, in the title of one of his last books, called 'the care of the self': that is, reflexive work upon the self in which individuals embed themselves in social practices, formulating new relationships to those practices in such a way as to have greater autonomy as well as more responsibility for the way these practices mould who they are. Group analysis itself could, in a similar spirit, be seen as a civilising process in which members of a group weave a matrix of communication that holds the group together and through which they learn to relate to each other, working through the fantasised transferential perceptions they have of each other.

All this, the clinical practice that promised to be a thoroughly social approach to psychoanalysis, together with a social theory that was close enough to Foucault to reflexively and historically embed itself in history as a political practice, was what led me in 1996 to the Institute of Group Analysis in Daleham Gardens, NW3. I sat facing Adele Mittwoch and, by her side, Ray Haddock, a young psychiatrist who I usually referred to as 'fish-face' after the two signifiers that comprise his name, and who had already given me a hard time in a psychiatric assessment during a meeting in Sheffield as part of my application for the IGA training. Behind the interview panel were what were known among group analysts as 'Michael's curtains', totemic heavy cloth items with gruesome scenes of Persian soldiers beheading captives. I couldn't see the scenes clearly, and neither could Michael.

The story was that, when Foulkes bought them from Liberty's department store in London for his group analytic practice, he only saw the pleasing general pattern, overlooking the violent detail. Michael's curtains were a running motif in some of the discussions about the difference between the relatively benign practice of group analysis and the more conflict-focused approaches of the followers of Bion and the Kleinians at the Tavistock Clinic just around the corner in Belsize Lane. But maybe Adele was right. I liked the approach, but my application had been rather precipitous, and there were a number of complications, the kind of complications that group analysts were very attuned to.

Median

We had travelled up to Monsall Hospital in north Manchester together every Thursday afternoon for a year in the early 1990s, during Operation Desert Shield and Operation Desert Storm and their aftermath, during protests against US imperialist intervention in Iraq, and bitter recrimination about the consequences. I have mentioned her, but I haven't really introduced Erica Burman yet in this narrative, but she is crucial to this part of the story so you should know who she is. Erica was a critical developmental psychologist, another anti-psychologist with a background in cognitive studies and artificial intelligence, who was in Manchester when I arrived there in 1985, and she was then a member of the psychology department at the Poly from 1986. She was active in radical mental health politics as a member of Mind in Manchester, and together we attended the Gaskell House Monday morning seminars, both going on to work as honorary psychotherapists. When I went down to the NELP Psychoanalysis and the Public Sphere conference in 1987 I stayed the night in Erica's sister's house. Friends would joke that we were a unit, the unit in the Discourse Unit research group we set up, it was an open secret that we were partners in the department, and so during the introductory course in group analysis at Monsall Hospital we were placed in separate groups.

Everything was 'group' here. The interview for the course in July 1990, which was a stand-alone and preliminary course for the IGA training and for the NWIDP training in Manchester, was at the Red House in Salford – the Red House was both a twin and a sometime rival NHS psychotherapy centre to Gaskell House. Gaskell House focused on individuals, and the Red House was the centre for group psychotherapy. The interview was in a group. No Erica because we had already declared our relationship on the application form. Six applicants were brought together for an hour by course convenor Keith Hyde, a softly-spoken psychiatrist with bad shirts, the kind with collars in a different colour shade, and a habit of smiling while he muttered, which meant you had to concentrate very hard to hear what he was saying. Keith was one of the good guys, something we were to learn later from radical political activists in distress who he had taken in for psychotherapy. At the time I was just frightened of him because he was a psychiatrist. The letter inviting me for interview said that 'we would like to meet you in a small group'.

The interview began with a long silence, which was eventually broken by one of the other applicants saying that he supposed that we should say who we were and talk about why we wanted to take the course. Keith smiled and nodded, so we did too, we introduced ourselves. Later on Keith asked us if we had any specific questions about the course, and one guy blurted out that he wanted to know whether it was possible to withdraw from the course before it started, because, he said, he had applied for things and done that before, withdrawn. We all looked at him, and glanced quickly at each other, each, I guess, thinking that we would not see this guy on the course, and so we didn't. That was that.

From 4 October 1990, Erica and I drove up to Monsall together after I had made soup, my early afternoon task. The course, run by the IGA in London and the North West Regional Health Authority, was the fourteenth course, and was in the NWRHA Staff College in the old isolation hospital for communicable diseases, very appropriate, the grounds of which were laid out like a film set with a faux village green and telephone box, and a corner building. This cloistered corner building was where we were able to take a break from our lecturing day jobs, able to be students again. Tea and coffee and biscuits were already there for students mingling after their own 'experiential small group', the group-analytic therapy component of the course. For us, in the second shift, the day started at 4.45 for an hour-long lecture or seminar group or 'experiential large group', then a break and then our ninety-minute experiential small group, the therapy group. Then we would drive home and eat the soup and watch *Star Trek: The Next Generation* I had video-recorded ready for our therapeutic wind-down from our group therapy day out. Therapy-speak was really starting to bloom in the wider culture by now, as evidenced in the role accorded to Deanna Troi as ship's counsellor on the Enterprise.

When there were lectures in the first session, these would be on topics like 'general principles of psychotherapy' given by Frank Margison, or 'what is therapeutic in a group' given by Terry Lear. That one was run on classic 'guess what is in my mind' teaching lines where we had to generate a list of factors important in running a group before Lear unrolled the flip chart to tell us what we had got right and what we had missed out. One time we had a guest lecture by Dorothy Stock Whitaker, who had written the course book *Using Groups to Help People*, an infuriatingly vague account of what happens in groups. When there were seminar groups after the break, mine were led by Bill Barnes, who was Erica's experiential small-group conductor, and when there were experiential large groups these were led by Anne Harrow.

The large groups included half the students who had already had their experiential small groups and were ready to go home. The talk among students in the breaks invariably turned to whether they would be taking the IGA training or the NWIDP training as their next step. These tea breaks were usually excruciating occasions, places where people from the same small groups studiously avoided each other, for to talk together outside the group might be interpreted as 'acting out'; the simple question 'how are you' would often be met by protracted silence and then a careful, drawn-out description of physical and mental states. These were places for the rehearsal and performance of therapeutic discourse in which students configured themselves as dutiful psychoanalytic subjects. If you didn't cry, you should at least be ready to acknowledge that there were feelings bubbling away beneath the surface that sometimes brought you close to the edge. There were a few academics, but most were nurses or other NHS care workers, many of whom were already running groups. For them, this was top-up in-service training. Most of the students were women.

The large groups were in a block of four weeks in January 1991, and were a political battleground. The 'coalition of the willing' was moving into the combat phase of the Gulf War, and opponents had mobilised against it in mass demonstrations, some of the largest the country had seen. Anne Harrow began the first large group by reminding us that a large group in group analysis is a group in which not everyone can be seen by the other participants, and so it was in this long raggedy room with perhaps seventy or so students and group convenors. It wasn't actually a very large group, perhaps it was what would in group-analytic terms be seen as a 'median' group. It was not really a large group, just as, we were sometimes reminded, our therapy groups were really only 'experiential small groups'. The 'aim' of the large group was glossed in the course brochure as being 'to experience the implications on individual functioning of the size of the group'. Anne suggested that we think of the large group as like society and our small experiential groups as like our family. "No," I said, unable to contain myself, "society is out there, where there is war and demonstrations against the war." For the next four weeks the talk revolved around the violence of war, with parallels being drawn between the occupation of territory in Kuwait and Iraq and the way that we might react if someone took our chair in the group and how we might defend it. It was enraging and compelling.

I think Sheila was amused. She sometimes looked amused. Sheila Ernst was the conductor of my experiential small group, and was Erica's seminar group leader. Sheila was the co-ordinator for group therapy and training at the Women's Therapy Centre in London, and had co-edited, with Marie Maguire, the 1987 volume *Living With the Sphinx: Papers From the Women's Therapy Centre*. Before that she had co-authored, with Lucy Goodison, a 1981 feminist classic *In Our Own Hands: A Book of Self-Help Therapy*. Sheila was one of the most important socialist-feminist activists in the 'second wave' of feminism of the 1960s and 1970s. She had gone into therapy as a place to work as a result of the implications of the second-wave feminist argument that 'the personal is political'. It was a generational shift into therapy, something that troubled me as a possible shift away from activism, and many of those feminist activists chose group analysis as the modality of therapy best suited to their political project, something that impressed me. The ethos of the course, and perhaps of group analysis overall was, I would say, progressive, and the co-authorship of an *Introduction to Groupwork* by Bill Barnes, Sheila Ernst and Keith Hyde was further evidence, if I needed it, that there was some political kinship between those running things that year at Monsall Hospital.

I so wanted Sheila to say feminist things in my group. She didn't say anything that explicitly, so I had to search for signs that she was conducting the group in a feminist or socialist way, or both, but then again, as during my individual therapy, I had little to go on. There were eleven of us in my group, including a much older academic who referred to books he had read about group analysis, a mistake that was ruthlessly interpreted as an academic defence mechanism, intellectualisation. A younger psychiatrist made the mistake one day of referring to 'strong northern women'; the strong northern women leant forward waggling their shoulders and stared at him. He blushed and shut up. My mistake was to casually mention one day that I wondered what would happen in the group if I hanged myself in the toilets. This was clearly a terrible thing to say, insensitive, thoughtless, and I was told so. I clearly mistook free associative play in the matrix of the group for uncivilized outbursts, for gabbling about whatever came into my mind.

Sheila's mistake in one session was to interpret the presence of herself and the psychiatrist as forming a social link, a supposed identity between the two of them. Small groups in the group analysis tradition are composed, Foulkes says, of at least two members of each identity group, with the exception of Jews. While it would not be a good idea to have only one man or only one woman or only one gay or only one lesbian in a group, he says, a single Jew already has sufficient experience of being isolated to be able to cope. Foulkes was Jewish and Norbert Elias, who was also a Jew, was gay, though not out, and it was difficult to know what was being played out in these statements about the composition of groups. Anyway, Sheila said, one day, that it was strange that no one had commented on the interaction between her and the psychiatrist, that they were both Jewish. The poor guy blushed again, and said that, no, he was not Jewish. We all laughed. Sheila laughed. The mistake didn't count against her, perhaps because we all knew how important she was and admired her too much.

I so wanted Sheila Ernst to notice me, another radical, that's why I wanted her to at least be amused by my outbursts about the war in the large group. I had to wait until another occasion, a year later in Manchester, at a conference, when an IPA psychoanalyst Peter Hildebrand gave an awful, reactionary paper about gay men and HIV/AIDS linking homosexuality with their illness. I objected publicly in the discussion, and was told by another psychotherapist, Lisa Herzog from Gaskell House, that my reaction was part of a general anxiety about death. Sheila came up to Erica and me in the break and said to me "I thought it would be you." I loved this. I interpreted this to myself as the recognition by another as a comrade that I had craved in the small group for a year.

Small

Psychoanalytic psychotherapy in Britain is a small, entangled world of personal-political relationships and rivalries. Sheila Ernst, for example, was married in the 1960s to Bob Young at *Free Associations*. We often encountered the criss-crossing paths of people we admired, sometimes role models, and the gossip about who had been in analysis with whom was a staple of distracted conversation around the edges of seminars and conferences.

By the end of 1995 I had finished seeing my patient at Gaskell House, finished with Don, my Anna Freudian therapist. Group analysis seemed the thing. Erica and I carried on attending the Friday seminars in Manchester, which brought together trainees on the diploma and outsiders like us. We attended psychoanalytic conferences, like the one with Hildebrand, saw Dorothy Stock Whitaker speak again on one of the IGA Fridays, started our short course 'Freudian foundations' at the Poly, and announced the master's in psychoanalytic studies would run there.

I had already given another paper, back in December 1993 at the Gaskell House meetings, on Bion's basic assumptions, to make sense of reactions in my department to staff sleeping with students. Fight-flight avoidance and anger by colleagues, dependency on the head of department to solve the problem, and bizarre displacement in attempts to pin the blame on pairing between two members of staff –Erica and me – were all in the mix. I tried to embed a psychoanalytic account of what was happening in an analysis of psychoanalytic culture, culture in which psychoanalytic discourse was used to make sense of disturbing phenomena.

A complicated chain of circumstances – a possible academic year abroad that meant I could not begin training in 1996, and then an academic post outside Manchester that meant I could – led to a tangle that the IGA had to assess and unravel. Erica and I met with a rather bemused Keith Hyde at the Red House to discuss whether it would be possible for us both to train with the IGA at the same time. He was understandably non-committal. Why, but why not? Erica applied to begin the IGA training to start in autumn 1996, and was accepted. I applied, first intending to defer for a year, that is, to begin in autumn 1997, and then changed my mind when I realised I would still be in the UK, and pressed ahead. Well, it was even more chaotic than that. Erica remembers me applying for CFAR at the same time. Fish-face probably thought I was crazy, or at least that this was a hare-brained scheme, not sure about what I was doing.

A part of me did want to do the group analysis training, especially so as Erica was going to do it, even if I also wondered if it was the right thing for me. Most importantly, at the time, I wanted to do it *now*, start as soon as possible. The IGA Training Committee probably made the right decision when they finally wrote to me in July to say that I had been accepted, good, but that 'your partner entering the same cohort … would not be in the best interests of your training'. Damn. They would let me in the following year, 1997. Too late, impatient Ian thought, as he manfully, with great restraint, folded up the letter again instead of crumpling it up.

Lacan talks about haste, and does so in relation to groups, in one of his few attempts to develop a theory of the social as such – another was in his account of the 'four discourses' that structure the social bonds that make psychoanalysis itself possible. More on the four discourses later. Lacan visited England after the Second World War and met Bion and Rickman, and he wrote a favourable report of their work at Northfield on his return to Paris. His theoretical foray into group dynamics came at around the same time in a paper on 'logical time', which was, among other things, a riposte to Sartre's assertion that hell is other people. No,

Lacan argued, you need other people to be human, to become a subject. In his 'logical time' paper, Lacan describes how three prisoners are invited to puzzle about who they are in relation to their fellow lags and to give an account of themselves to the warder. Whereupon, if they are successful, they will be released. What they see and what they know is conditioned by how they see and when they hesitate, and what they make of the others' hesitation as they too try to make sense of who they are. Your relation to others, a relation that Lacan did at that time conceptualise as being 'intersubjective', is bound up with your relationship to time. Time again. I had seen what I needed to of group analysis, and what I knew of it was connected to how others in that tradition of work related to me. I made a break for it, looking for a way out, and you have had enough clues so far to know where this led me.

10

PERSONAL

Training analysis

I fell among the Lacanians. I describe here how I applied for training, and went deeper into analysis as a prerequisite for beginning the course. This chapter is about the first key component of a training course, and here I try to make sense of the relationship between institutional requirements and the demand for analysis, between the desire to become an analyst and the need to undergo treatment.

Rules

In 1920, when the IPA had around 200 members, Max Eitingon organised a system of training through the Berlin Training Commission at the Berlin Polyclinic. The Eitingon Training Model, sometimes known as the Berlin Model or Berlin Rules, had three components: training analysis, theoretical instruction, and supervision of analytic cases. Even at that time, many psychoanalysts had not undergone psychoanalysis themselves, a couple of meetings with Freud sometimes sufficed, as was the case for his favourite, Wilhelm Reich. There was no formal series of lectures for trainees, and supervision was not the norm. Freud himself declared once that anyone who recognises transference and resistance is a psychoanalyst, is, as he put it, part of 'our mad horde'. An International Training Commission was set up in 1925 to regularise training, and this tripartite system has been the standard model for psychoanalysts in different organisations around the world ever since.

This model was also adopted by the Lacanians in Britain when they developed their own clinical training organisation. A Cultural Centre for Freudian Studies and Research had been set up by Bice Benvenuto, Bernard Burgoyne, Richard Klein and Darian Leader immediately after the 1985 Cambridge conference I described in Chapter 3. The following year Jacques-Alain Miller spoke at a 'Lacan in England' conference, and insisted that all the other speakers should be explicitly affiliated with his own École de la cause freudienne, or approved by him. So it was that the

Centre's newsletter, *Syngraphia*, announced itself as 'the enunciation of the CCFSR from within the Champ-Freudian, from within the field of the Other'. The editorials by Richard Klein in the Centre's journal in the early 1990s were no less mysterious, as you would expect. By now the organisation had rebranded itself as the Centre for Freudian Analysis and Research, CFAR (say it 'see far'). The first issue of the *Journal of the Centre for Freudian Analysis and Research*, in 1992, declared that 'between Freud and Lacan there is one straight line', and signalled its affiliation to Miller's World Association of Psychoanalysis, a Lacanian alternative to the IPA.

In some ways there could be no bigger difference between training organisations than between the IGA, the Institute of Group Analysis, and CFAR. The IGA was determinedly therapeutic, bringing together psychoanalytic psychotherapists from different traditions of work, including Jungians, who liked to think of the matrix as a place where archetypes circulated, and even followers of Bion and the Kleinian tradition, who conducted their groups within the frame of the Tavistock tradition. The IGA even included advocates of alternative systemic therapies that were not psychoanalytic at all, though there weren't, as far as I knew, any Lacanians involved.

CFAR, on the other hand, was avowedly psychoanalytic, insisting that although psychoanalysis has what they called 'therapeutic effects', this was not the primary aim of the treatment, and their recondite formulations in the journal seemed designed to keep outsiders at bay, even to warn them off in sectarian reminders that the Centre was with Jacques-Alain Miller as the voice of Lacan on Earth. This Millerian stance had softened a bit by 1997, by which time *JCFAR* had included an article by Slavoj Žižek, admittedly at that time an acolyte of Miller, and by Yannis Stavrakakis, a student of Ernesto Laclau who, with Chantal Mouffe, took up Žižek and promoted him in the English-speaking world. The Millerians were also beginning to organise separately from CFAR in the London Circle, which they founded in 1994.

Genie Georgaca, who finished her PhD in 1996, was by now well into the CFAR training. Erica began her IGA training that autumn as planned. I was a little jealous, felt left out. I could have joined the IGA training in autumn 1997, a year below Erica, but I was still unsure which was, which is, the most thoroughly 'social' version of psychoanalysis. On the one hand, in its theory and practice, group analysis was social in the sense that everything was mediated by the group, though it is true that Foulkes did characterise the approach as 'ego training in action'. On the other hand, Lacan had, in theory, shifted focus to language such that, as one southern-state US friend's formulation had it, 'everything goes through the Other', though in practice the clinical practice was still one-to-one, one by one.

There were intriguing group elements to Lacanian work, in Lacan's theorisation of collective work in training in the new school of psychoanalysis he set up in 1964, for example. The signifier 'research' was also important to CFAR, and it wanted to forge connections between artisans and theorists using psychoanalysis in academic and cultural projects, not only to train clinical practitioners. To speak not only of the unconscious as 'structured like a language' but also of the unconscious as 'the discourse of the Other' connected with Marxist political theory of the kind elaborated by Ernesto Laclau and Chantal Mouffe.

These people used Lacanian theory, but I was starting to realise that this social theory was very different from a theoretical underpinning of Lacanian psychoanalytic clinical practice. At a 1995 meeting in Manchester, organised by the Human Sciences seminar in the Poly, for example, Chantal Mouffe retreated into crass, mass-psychological explanations for group conflict, asserting that she thought Žižek was right in his claim that there was something in human nature that drove people to identify with different communities and then come into conflict with each other. I was very surprised, having read Žižek as saying exactly the opposite, or, as he would probably have put it, 'precisely the reverse', that our identification with different groups is socially structured and that our sense of individual identity is felt at depth by us as an illusion, individual identity as 'the sublime object' of ideology.

Žižek's melange of Lacan, Marx and Hegel in *The Sublime Object of Ideology* also had something to do with the shift I was making, from an interest in group analysis to wanting to know more about Lacan. What to make of Žižek was another matter. I came away from his books reeling, unable to explain what I had read to my friends. We organised a meeting in the Discourse Unit with Antony Easthope to describe and discuss Žižek, but were none the wiser afterwards. Genie said that Antony didn't understand Žižek either.

Regulations

The only way to find out about Lacanian psychoanalysis, I decided, would be to immerse myself in it, and so I pursued my application for the CFAR training, and had my first interview on 1 July 1997, a year after I had received the IGA letter deferring my entry onto their diploma course. I travelled to and from London that Tuesday, a journey into Euston from Manchester and a gloomy walk along Euston Road to St Pancras, where I took a local train up to Elstree and Borehamwood for a meeting with Gillian Darcy. Gloomy, as I pondered again the relationship between politics and psychoanalysis and what I was doing, contemplating plunging into years of training that would seriously sidetrack me from activism, from other kinds of meetings.

The IGA training was based in Manchester under the auspices of GAN, Group Analysis North, and ran on a 'block weekend' basis about once a month, with a Friday seminar, the Friday events we had already attended, followed by groups from Friday evening through Saturday and Sunday – and that included the therapy groups. This would be more manageable, I thought, than travelling to London every Saturday for the CFAR lectures and seminars. I went into Housmans, a radical bookshop near King's Cross, which made me feel worse, guiltier. When I got to her house, Gillian asked me what I thought was the most important concept in Lacanian theory. I talked about discourse and the unconscious before she reminded me of the correct answer, posed as a tentative question inviting me to agree, "lack?".

Lack in Lacanian theory is not quite the same as therapeutic 'disappointment' that you need, according to some conservative authors, to come to terms with, but it does call for acceptance of the inevitability, for all those who speak, of castration by the signifier. Yes, that's what 'castration' is for Lacanians: not the chopping off of your willy but subjection to the limits imposed by language, the Law of the Symbolic, what is sometimes rather infelicitously referred to as the 'Name of the Father'. Even if you don't always choose your words carefully, you always choose your words, and there are many times when you are repeating what has been said about you or to you: your words choose you, limit you. In a first approach to lack as close to buckling under to disappointment, you come to terms with the fact you won't always get what you want and you limit your desires accordingly. This might have been what Foucault had in mind when he shouted out, during one of Lacan's seminars, "I do not lack!". Here is a key conceptual difference between Lacan and psychotherapy; lack should also be thought of as closely linked to the nature of language itself rather than to 'feelings' that you sense should be expressed. It can be thought of as that missing tile in the child's 'sliding puzzle', the space that enables the other letters to move around. There is a real problem when there is a lack of a lack, then you really are stuck.

The first rule of the Lacan club was analysis, so I moved fast. There were few Lacanian psychoanalysts in Britain, even if you combined those who had graduated from the CFAR training, who numbered around twenty, and analysts from abroad who had trained elsewhere. This was a small pool to choose from, even if you took into account that a majority of psychoanalysts in the world were now either directly trained in a Lacanian framework or had moved over from their initial IPA-organisation training to Lacan. You had to go outside the English-speaking world to find these analysts, and many of them were in the Latin-language countries, particularly in Latin America, and their absence from the scene in Britain made it easier for the British Psychoanalytical Society to pretend that Lacanian clinical work simply didn't exist. This was one reason why CFAR did not stipulate that the training analysis should necessarily be with a Lacanian. Candidates may have already been in analysis with a psychoanalyst from another tradition when they decided to train. More important than that, although most Lacanians felt sore about the exclusion of Lacan from the IPA in 1963, by what he referred to as his 'excommunication', they did not go all the way with the argument that *only* Lacanian psychoanalysis was the real deal.

There were close contacts between Lacanians and IPA psychoanalysts in other parts of the world, even the existence of Lacanian groups inside the IPA, in Quebec, for example, where there was innovative radical work on 'psychosis'. And when Lacan insisted that he was engaging in a 'return to Freud', this was often read as a return to a close reading not only of Freud's texts but also of the texts of the different traditions of work that had appeared after Freud's death. Lacanians recognised IPA members as psychoanalysts, of course, and it was in their interests to support any initiatives that valued a plurality of perspectives as part of the broad field of Freudian work.

The field of possible analysts was much smaller for me because I was in Manchester, and I was not going to go into analysis with Kleinian John, even if he had agreed to have me. There was no one else around. The field was not as narrow as it could have been, however, because of a principled difference between the IPA and Lacanian traditions. It was a difference that flowed partly from the conditions in which Lacan was excommunicated and partly from his critique of the bureaucratisation of the IPA. The IPA training relied on the work of the 'training analysts', that is a higher caste of analyst, senior, older, who were also much more likely to be medically trained.

The requirement that one must be in analysis with a 'training analyst' in order for it to be recognised as a 'training analysis' seemed to Lacan to be a travesty of psychoanalysis as such. This requirement reinforced the vertically-organised hierarchical basis of the IPA globally and of each separate component organisation. This was the situation still in Britain where the training analyst was expected to report to the training committee on the progress of the candidate, a situation that, as we already have seen, had disastrous consequences for gay men or lesbians who had committed to training after keeping quiet about their sexuality during the application interviews. CFAR had no such expectation. Precisely the reverse; one's personal analysis was that, personal, necessary but also sacrosanct. You could go as mad in your own analysis as you liked.

The requirement that analysis must be with someone already designated as a 'training analyst', who would thereby guarantee that things were running on the right track, also ran counter to an authentically psychoanalytic conception of time. Time again. This time, it was training that needed to be conceptualised as operating *Nachträglich*, after the event, *après coup*. A tranche of psychoanalysis could only be considered to be a training analysis after the event, in retrospect, when the analysand had made a decision, was subject to the act of becoming a psychoanalyst. This became linked to the Lacanian dictum that the only authorisation of a psychoanalyst comes from the psychoanalyst themselves. This is not to say that the context for that authorisation and self-authorisation is unimportant, but it is to insist that a psychoanalyst is not merely made by a committee decision or through the giving of a label by a group or an institution. There is much more to it than that. CFAR warned that psychoanalysis may also provide the context for a candidate who had been accepted for training on its course to decide that they did not want to become a psychoanalyst after all.

I tracked down an Argentinian colleague of Genie's analyst. Argentinian was good, very good. Argentina has the highest concentration of Lacanian psychoanalysts in the world, and a reputation for exporting high-power theorists around the world. Ernesto Laclau was Argentinian, for example. Amelia Mangani lived in Chester, not too far from Manchester, and I arranged an appointment to see her at her house the following Wednesday. I told Amelia when I saw her that I wanted to start the CFAR training and admitted that this was not in itself a good enough reason to begin analysis. She seemed to agree. I said I wasn't even really sure why I wanted to do the training, but I wanted to find out about Lacan. I remembered John Churcher's account of his successful application interview for training at the

Institute of Psychoanalysis. The panel had asked him why he wanted to train as a psychoanalyst and he said he didn't know. It was a smart, but risky, reply. I said to Amelia that I wasn't sure about all the travelling, train travel that would really turn the course into training, including travelling every week to Chester, but no, I said, "I'm only joking". Amelia replied, ending our meeting, with quite a good interpretation that rang in my ears on the way back to the station, "maybe you are joking yourself?". What on earth did that mean? Anyway, we had another appointment set up to get things underway at her office in the centre of Chester. There was no couch in the room. We sat face-to-face.

The Thursday after my first meeting with Amelia I was back to London again for my second CFAR interview, this time a trek down and across to Liverpool Street station, to 'Just Ask Counselling and Advisory Service' to meet with Gerry Sullivan. It seemed a strange institutional context to talk about Lacanian psychoanalysis, which relies, I had read, on the analysand making a 'demand' for analysis, not just asking, and I knew that Lacanians would not give advice. We chatted about discourse and Laclau and Mouffe for a bit, and Gerry said he knew of the journal *Ideology and Consciousness*, in which I had first read articles about Lacan in the late 1970s. I told him I had begun analysis. When? Last week. This was a problem, he said. What?

CFAR was accredited as a training organisation with the UKCP, the United Kingdom Council for Psychotherapy, which has over 8,000 members registered, and so the organisation needed to abide by UKCP rules, which stipulated that a candidate must be in therapy for at least one year prior to beginning the training and then throughout the training. This was Berlin Rules with a bite. There was no way round it, Gerry said, and he was surprised Gillian hadn't mentioned this at my first interview. Lack. Castration. Disappointment. Gerry said he would take the discussion we had back to the training committee, and that I should wait for a year, contact CFAR to have one more interview so they were updated on my progress, and then it should not be a problem to start in autumn 1998. 1998! Another year!

I dutifully carried on with my personal analysis with Amelia, occasionally railing against the requirement that I be in analysis. There should be a demand for analysis, I complained, not something that should be enforced. I didn't want to be in analysis as a condition for starting the training. I wanted to be in analysis as something I had chosen because I wanted to be in analysis. Such complaint could, of course, be easily interpreted as my resistance to what was being uncovered in the analysis, and Amelia did not need to tell me that. My frustration was, at the very least, something to talk about in Chester, and, I eventually heard myself making connections between my descriptions of that particular situation and other earlier significant times of my life. The sessions were not on a fixed day. Amelia would tell me when she could see me the following week, which was also something to talk about, something to complain about. This became something of a running joke between Erica and me, one of the marked differences between her time in the analytic groups on the block weekends and my own sessions with Amelia. Group analysis made a big deal about what they called 'dynamic administration', the careful organisation of the analytic space, attention to context, and the concern with avoiding, wherever possible, extraneous events or disruptions to the routine of the analysis.

As with the quasi-Winnicottian psychoanalytic psychotherapy I had conducted at Gaskell House, group analysts would always comment upon breaks in that routine, drawing attention to them, anticipating any possible disturbance, any possible effect on the transference, interpreting that transference. Lacanians, on the other hand, seemed to treat such things as something to talk about. If the analysand wanted to talk about it, all well and good, but analysis was, in this respect, treated as something that happened in the clinic as part of the world. In Erica's own analysis before she started the GAN training, for example, her analyst told her once that the following week there would be something different in the room. A couch arrived.

Disruptions

One day a couch arrived in the corner of Amelia's office. I wanted to lie on it, wanted this to turn into a proper analysis. "Proper analysis," Amelia chuckled. "You want to do it properly" – an allusion to a signifier I had used to describe how shitting had been talked about in my family. Very amusing. I said that in your own personal analysis you could go as mad as you liked, but that wasn't strictly true. If there was a danger of you going mad, then a Lacanian would not let you on the couch. Gerry Sullivan had referred to this during my application interview at 'Just Ask'. "Once a week," he said, when I was trying to reassure him that I had already begun analysis and that it would be two, almost three months before the CFAR training began that year. "Well, twice a week has quite different effects to once a week, and I've seen people go quite mad on the couch." I must admit, and it won't surprise you, that I was frightened of going mad. I was frightened of psychiatrists, so that was reason enough to be frightened of going mad.

Lacan said that no one could go mad of their own volition, but I wondered if I could go mad if I thought about it or talked about it too much, that something like that could happen in analysis. I had an image of dropping down the edge of a deep slide, the kind you find in a funfair where you momentarily lose consciousness as you fall and open your eyes at the bottom of the drop where you are lying on your back. Perhaps to really engage in 'free association' in analysis would be the same. I was careful about what I said, too careful most of the time. Amelia's couch looked at me from the corner of the room, and I felt annoyed that she wasn't inviting me to lie down there, to move on from these prolonged 'preliminary sessions'. I knew that the stretch of preliminary sessions tended to be much longer in Lacanian psychoanalysis, with judgements made by the analyst as to whether the analysand was psychotic, that the preliminary sessions were characterised by attention to the possible existence of what was called 'psychotic structure'. Did Amelia think I was mad? Eventually I persuaded her that I was not, or I gave up trying to persuade her that I was not mad, and then it was time to move onto the couch. But then, wait a minute, time's up! These were variable length sessions.

The notice I had to give for missing sessions was less than it had been for Don, now twenty-four hours, but the timing of the sessions was more, well, erratic. I felt it as erratic, and sometimes as calculated. It wasn't long before I got the message from CFAR that candidates were really expected to be in analysis at least twice a week, and so that's what I arranged with Amelia, and she said that these two sessions could be on the same day, which meant that I only needed to make one trip to Chester a week. During her time in the centre of Chester this was by train. I would travel down, usually in the morning, and have a session. Amelia would tell me to come back later, which, if I was lucky, would give me time to have a cup of tea and a sandwich in a nice café on the high street. If I was unlucky, it would be too short a time to do that and I would walk around the city walls for a while, and, if I was really unlucky, this would be an evening visit and the café would be closed, it would be dark, it would be raining.

Then Amelia moved to the outskirts of the city, and I began to travel by car. Here, she didn't have a couch, but I sat in a kind of garden deck chair. She sat behind me. The couch itself was not the psychoanalytic device. The relationship or lack of relation was the device. It meant I could not look for clues as to what she was thinking, for how she responded to what I was saying, to my jokes and complaints. Instead, I listened to myself speak, focused on the flow of words or, more, so the breaks and gaps between them. What I heard myself say surprised me, and shook me from assumptions I had often made about who I was and who I should be. I was teaching in Bolton, north-west of Manchester, and would then race down the motorway on Monday evenings for a session at 6.30. If things went to plan I could have a session, then sit in the car for about fifteen minutes to listen to *The Archers*, 'an everyday story of country folk' serial on BBC Radio 4, go back for the second session at 7.15, and finish in time to go to the nearby supermarket to do the weekly shopping, arriving back after the forty-minute drive to Manchester for a late dinner. It didn't always go to plan.

Unlike the sessions with Don, which had run in line with the standard fifty-minute hour, Amelia's sessions were around thirty minutes long, sometimes hardly time enough, I thought, to get started on a detailed description of something that had happened in my childhood, sometimes too long to bear. I spent some sessions almost in complete silence, wondering how long she would put up with this, but I would crack first and speak; after all I was paying for this time, and now wasting it. Occasionally the sessions were longer than half an hour, but usually they were quite a deal less. When that happened and she told me to come back fifteen minutes later I would miss *The Archers* altogether, though listening to it in the break was always my secret, something I never told her about. How I managed time and kept secrets was as much a part of the analysis as what I said; I noticed what I was doing and repeated what I did in different contexts with a different awareness of what it meant to me as I related to others.

My calculations over the use of the time never seemed to coincide completely with what Amelia was doing with it, and sometimes I longed for the routine that seemed to mark Freud's own regular-length sessions in Vienna, the fifty minutes that became the benchmark of the thoroughly formalised Berlin Rules. I knew that those fifty-minute blocks of time were themselves an artifice, a function of the architecture of Freud's apartment and of his family life. Martha, his wife, had commented once when she was showing a visitor, Melitta Schmideberg, around the apartment that she liked to water the plants in the consulting room every hour, and needed about ten minutes to do so thoroughly. Melitta Schmideberg, a psychoanalyst herself, Melanie Klein's daughter, deduced from this that the fifty minutes available between Martha's plant-waterings thus became the basis of standard analytic practice.

Amelia would sometimes cut the session at ten minutes. Very Argentinian, I thought. Sometimes I would try to speak to her in Spanish and she would ask, in Spanish, "Por que acá?". Why here? Good question. Was I trying to impress her by speaking her language, show some affiliation with her, identification even, or was it an alternative to speaking the language of analysis itself, which I wasn't even sure I should be doing? I had heard that ten-minute sessions were the practice of some Lacanian psychoanalysts in Argentina, a practice that really did turn Freudian analysis into something different, into so-called 'short sessions'. No, what Amelia was doing was in line with Lacanian 'variable-length sessions', which were based, once again, on a psychoanalytic theory of time. Variable-length sessions enable the psychoanalyst to mark a particular point as significant without offering a laborious 'interpretation' that spells out exactly what was meant by a hesitation, a slip of the tongue or the repetition of a signifier. To cut a session is thus to give an interpretation and, better, such an interpretation is ambiguous.

To cut a session in this way also opens up the time between the sessions as a time for the analysand to puzzle over the meaning of that particular cut. This is rather like the phenomenon that Bluma Zeigarnik, who was working in a phenomenological framework, noticed: unfinished tasks would be ruminated over, out of direct consciousness, and then only disappear when the task had been completed. To say that psychoanalysis can operate in line with the Zeigarnik effect would, Lacan commented, be to psychologise it, reduce what is happening to some internal cognitive process, but there is nonetheless something significant happening here. Such an interpretation seizes hold, has an effect, after the event, not at the moment the analyst decides to make it.

Interpretations seized me, but they did so after the event, and they were usually not interpretations that were sledgehammered home by my analyst until I got the point. They were, rather, interpretations that I was able to make myself, connections between signifiers that I had never made before, connections I was able to make because I attempted to speak freely and my struggle at free association was witnessed by another who was not sitting in judgement on my speech. There were moments of boredom, of frustration and of liberation, something that only that closed private space is able to provide. I had been schooled in a political tradition that treats public collective action as the space of liberation, but there are some things that can only be said and heard away from the world. The clinic is in the world but, in a strange way, not entirely of it. It is 'extimate' to it. I guess what I learned was not how fascinating I was to myself – that would be to configure psychoanalysis as the self-indulgent navel-gazing that opponents of touchy-feely hippy culture make it out to be – but rather how fascinating speech, as such, is, the language I spoke, using terms and phrases I could not entirely control, and the language I heard others use as they encountered the same and different cultural conditions that made them human beings. I never understood, for example, the complaint by Jeffrey Masson in his 1984 book *The Assault on Truth*. Masson became bored with psychoanalysis and moved on, lingering long enough to disparage a practice that never seemed to really grab him. Beyond and despite the stupid, internal wrangles between psychoanalysts there was something more important, the practice they dedicated themselves to and cherished and defended.

In this way, I was, at the very least, learning something about the practice of analysis and noticing its effects, even while I was champing at the bit, waiting for the thing to be over, not knowing when that would be, unable to predict or control the process, which would have been a rather mad thing to try to do. I was a bit mad to rush into psychoanalytic training, and I was perhaps a bit obsessional to hesitate and prevaricate about it for so long, and for sure I wailed like a hysteric about what I had let myself in for. For Lacanians, that is good, they 'hystericise' the analysand, incite them to rebel, and then make them think about where they are in the complaints they make. In some way, my desire to be a psychoanalyst was a symptom, something I was not yet cured of, if I ever would be. The psychoanalytic twist on the joke about one psychotherapist and the light bulb that wanted to change was that, no, we are all attached to our symptoms, the light bulb does not want to change. At least I had a better idea what I was doing, what I had done, by launching myself into this. This was the practice, theoretically-informed practice, so let us turn now to the second element of the Berlin model, theoretical instruction.

11

DIAGNOSIS

Clinical structures

Now we are deep into the CFAR training, returning to Freud with Lacan, but with some uncomfortable questions remaining about the relationship between psychoanalysis and psychiatry. In this chapter, I trace the development of Freud's differential diagnosis of neuroses, psychosis and perversion from psychiatry through to present-day psychoanalytic practice, and explore some of the dilemmas this poses for those who turn to analysis as an alternative to mainstream 'labels' for behaviour and experience. Along the way you will learn something about the madness of psychoanalytic training institutions.

Anomie

The chairs, so much was said about the chairs. I took the early morning train down to London on the last Saturday in September 1998, and then the tube to Chalk Farm. Up Haverstock Hill on the right is number 76, Rathbone Books, and in the cellar are the chairs. A narrow flight of steps behind the bookshop counter led down into a musty, low-ceilinged cellar, a long room with a concrete floor and with a room divider halfway back. Down around to the left was a table. The speaker sat behind it, and ranged back into the room there was space for seventy or eighty people if they pushed the metal, black fold-up chairs close together. Some people brought cushions, but even then the chair backs shot up at a weird angle, not for adults, and their hard seats transmitted the cold from the concrete up into the whole body. This is CFAR, the first session of the year. I had had a meeting with Vivien Bar in June that year to confirm that I was in analysis and wanted to take up a place on the training. This meeting was at her home near Turnpike Lane; the last time I had been there was for an anti-fascist demonstration. Now we are training. I have paid my £1,095 for the year, cheap compared with IPA training, but that does not include the cost of analysis, nor, when the time comes, supervision. We are in a cellar, but we are in NW3, just. There was a panel introduction to psychoanalysis late morning for two hours to the whole student group, and then the room dividers were concertinaed shut in the afternoon ready for a year one, group introduction to 'Freudian structures'.

I say it was a group. Erica laughed. She had already had the first block weekend in Manchester for the second year of her group analysis training. This was worse. While group analysis was underpinned by a sociological theory of the civilising process, described by Norbert Elias, and the small groups were devoted to an exploration of the members' actual and fantasised relationships with each other, the CFAR training was characterised more by what the sociologist Émile Durkheim called 'anomie', a pathological fragmentation of rules and values experienced by individuals as lack of moral guidance. There was a rudimentary course guide and a termly list of lectures, but no reading lists for sessions, nothing of the 'aims' and 'objectives' for sessions that had been laboriously spelt out in the IGA introductory course, and no invitation to find out who else was new on the course and why we were there. I'm complaining now. I complained then, to Erica.

But perhaps this was deliberate, this formal structure of the training that was designed to speak better of its content. CFAR spurned the therapeutic ethos of self-disclosure and sharing of feeling, and it scorned the academic apparatus of detailed instructions that usually had more the effect of infantilising students than simply providing information. On the very rare occasions when some reading was mentioned in the cellar beyond a text by Freud or Lacan, it was done with a shrug, as if the idea that we would all read the same thing was somehow distasteful. There was Oliver Rathbone's bookshop upstairs, which was linked to Karnac Books, and there was a library, the running of which we sometimes discussed in student meetings. There were matters to be taken to the 'Oikos' committee that was devoted to housekeeping arrangements. Londoners spent some time in the Haverstock Hill centre painting the place, or clearing up when the cellar was flooded. More often we moaned about the chairs that Bernard Burgoyne had bought cheaply, and sometimes this recrimination about the bad purchase spilled into his exasperated suggestion that anyone could look around for better chairs if they liked. I consulted homeware catalogues, found some details of cheap, comfy chairs but didn't know what to do with the information. I was invited by the Oikos committee to find funding for replacement chairs. I gave up.

Eventually I got to know the other seven trainees in my year group. We cautiously, tentatively, shared names and I slowly pieced together an idea of what they knew about Lacan and what they wanted to do with it. Most had some academic background either as master's students on one of the psychoanalytic studies courses that were starting to spring up around the country, or as teachers of psychoanalysis in one of the human sciences, and a couple were already working as counsellors or psychotherapists. The standard format for sessions was that the speaker would take up almost all of the time, and then there might be a question or two, and then people would stand for a break, rubbing their cold bums and their sore backs. Most lectures were to the whole group, and often there one or two members of CFAR sitting in the audience; even the 'introductory' lectures were rehearsing and extending pretty arcane ideas, and I started to realise that the narrative usually traced a detailed hermetic circuit from a first idea that had been signalled in the title of the lecture to some other ideas in Lacan via Freud and, if there was time, back again.

We were each assigned tutors, and we had to make contact with them to discuss our progress. We were told to do this once a term. One Saturday I managed to fit in some time with Lindsay Watson at CFAR, but after that would go to her apartment near Kentish Town for a brief meeting every three or four months. Lindsay should give the go-ahead for starting to think about taking on training cases, I was told. I would need to arrange for a supervisor and pay for that separately myself. And Lindsay would, when the time was right, discuss what I was preparing for papers to be presented to the training committee to complete the training: two theoretical essays and two clinical case studies.

Back to Haverstock Hill, where Janet Low, who had started the course before me, would either raise the question of the chairs again or get CFAR to say something publicly about contemporary events. I knew Janet had started before me because there was an internal bulletin assembled by the students, including by Janet who was an organiser. This bulletin was not for public consumption, and all the more interesting for that. When it arrived off the press and was distributed to us in the basement in Haverstock Hill from a carefully-guarded pack in a plastic bag, I felt like a real insider.

Halfway between Chalk Farm tube station and Rathbone Books there was a road sign mounted on two metal poles that straddled half the width of the pavement, about two feet apart. Every time I made the journey up to the bookshop on a Saturday morning I would deliberately walk between these poles, sometimes holding my breath. I imagined entering a wormhole in space-time, to another Lacanian universe, and sometimes tried to envisage stepping directly into another time at the end of the training, out of that universe. It was at times like this that times in analysis would flash into my mind and I would be transported into a different kind of space. It was as I stepped between the two poles, under the sign, that I looked up from the pavement to see the bookshop frontage and perhaps some of my fellow trainees standing outside drinking coffee or smoking.

Janet would repeatedly urge CFAR to issue statements giving psychoanalytic interpretations of political issues. This was coolly received, and she would complain bitterly when her papers for the training committee had been turned back that she must, as she put it, "be writing for the wrong big Other". I thought she was brave to insist on a political dimension to psychoanalysis, but I also thought this was the wrong way to go about it. It is one thing to speak about the politics of psychoanalysis, how our practice fitted into contemporary culture, but that was very different from reframing issues psychoanalytically, within psychoanalytic discourse. Then, I thought, we would be part of the problem rather than engaging in a political intervention.

This was a difference of approach that continued to rankle between us, and, more implicitly between me and those who had really been acculturated so thoroughly into psychoanalytic discourse that they treated psychoanalysis as a world view. Then, why not, you could characterise certain regimes according to different Freudian clinical structures. You could then, with Žižek, see Nazi Germany as psychotic because there was a paranoiac search for enemies, the Other of the Other pulling the strings behind the scenes, and see Stalinist Russia as perverse because the party turned itself into an object-instrument of the Other's jouissance as an instrument of history. Capitalism as such could be viewed as obsessional, concerned with prediction and control as an ideological strategy for coping with its endemic crises, and resistance would then amount to little more than hysterical complaint. In this way capitalism and anti-capitalist movements complemented each other, two sides of neurotic structure.

It was unclear where psychoanalytic politics, the crazy narcissism of small differences that were beginning to erupt inside Lacanian organisations, would fit with these uses of clinical structures as a guide to world politics. There was some delighted discussion in early sessions at CFAR in autumn 1998 of Otto Kernberg's critique of IPA training, an insider critique by the IPA president published in *The International Journal of Psychoanalysis* two years before called 'Thirty Methods to Destroy the Creativity of Psychoanalytic Candidates'. We could surely match the IPA on insider critique at least.

Our internal bulletin that autumn included details of the twenty-two current full members of CFAR and the different student year groups, many of whom were listed as in the 'continuation year' after years one, two and three, something that caused me some anxiety. I knew that the continuation year was a very long indeterminate stretch of time, and during all that time the student was required to be in analysis. The autumn 1998 CFAR bulletin included a rather startling article by Bernard Burgoyne, which fingered Richard Klein, one of the organisation's co-founders, as the author of a scurrilous, unsigned article in another Lacanian publication denouncing CFAR. Richard had ceded editorship of *JCFAR*, the *Journal for Freudian Analysis and Research*, to Marc Du Ry in 1994, and disappeared from the editorial team altogether the following year with the appearance of issue number 6, which included essays by Colette Soler, who was based in Paris, on the body, and by Paul Verhaeghe, who was based in Ghent, on neurosis and perversion. The third article, by the Argentinian Silvia Elena Tendlarz, was on autistic children. Tendlarz continued to be a loyal member of Jacques-Alain Miller's World Association of Psychoanalysis, of which the European School and then, as a third lowest institutional layer, the London Circle were components. Soler and Verhaeghe, however, were beginning to distance themselves from Miller, and would do so more explicitly in the years to come. Miller, as we know, demanded obedience, and the burden of Bernard Burgoyne's 1998 CFAR bulletin article, which was titled 'The Freudian Field in London', was clear.

Burgoyne defended CFAR's work as an organisation loyal to Miller, pointing out that England was one of the most difficult contexts in which to build a Lacanian organisation. 'This work,' Burgoyne pointed out, was not easy, 'was not,' as he put it, 'that of putting up a deckchair in a garden.' CFAR had maintained what he called 'supportive relations' with the London Circle, which now had over forty members, of which thirty were also members or students of CFAR. There was a joint programme of the 'Freudian Field seminars'. Burgoyne rebutted the claim made by Richard Klein that CFAR had 'sought to become legitimised by local politics', by which Klein clearly meant participation in the UKCP, the body that now required all CFAR trainees to be in analysis throughout the years of the course. Burgoyne pointed out that CFAR had been responsible for the withdrawal of the British Psychoanalytical Society from the UKCP, leaving CFAR as an influential organisation within it speaking for psychoanalysis, no mean feat for a Lacanian group. Richard Klein had implied that CFAR was quickly churning out badly trained psychoanalysts with a clinical training in which, he claimed, the existing members 'pass on their non-experience'. This was harsh, but it was also not reassuring, as a first-year trainee, to read Bernard Burgoyne reassuring the Paris leadership of the WAP, that is, Jacques-Alain Miller, that most people took six or seven years or that some even took over ten years.

It is true that there was a large overlap between membership of CFAR as a more open, eclectic Lacanian organisation and the London Circle as a Millerian group. It was starting to dawn on me that Miller's 'international', the WAP, was not the only international network, and CFAR was keen to welcome Lacanians from around the world who came from different discrete traditions. Soon there was to be another network, another international, with the departure of Colette Soler at a 1998 conference in Barcelona organised under the auspices of Miller's École de la cause freudienne, the ECF, inherited from Lacan. The ECF had been set up by Lacan in 1981, after the dissolution of his existing school, shortly before he died. Colette Soler took out about a third of the members in 1998 to set up her own group, after Miller had tried to clamp down on dissenting voices in the ECF, declaring that if anyone had a problem they could come to talk to him about it 'one by one', as he put it.

Ripples from this split in the ECF rippled through the basement over the following months. Richard Klein had clearly signalled his loyalty to Miller, and saw the London Circle as the place to be. He resigned from CFAR, and sharper divisions between the two groups started to appear, either in the disappearance of some members and even trainees from the cellar, or in heated discussion between the breaks over what was going on. Heather Menzies, a graduate of the Kent psychoanalytic studies programme, who was now in the 'continuation year', for example, was most irritated after one talk in which the speaker reported that Miller had recently announced at a meeting in Paris that he had been told things by Lacan that he had not yet revealed. Miller had claimed in a bizarre metaphorical turn of phrase, for someone who was Jewish yet taking the leadership of the ECF from his father-in-law, raised a Catholic, that he, Miller, was "the pound of flesh of the thought of Jacques Lacan". This is destructive, stupid gossip, Heather said afterwards, as a small group of us clustered around her to hear her side of the story. "They are all Marxists in Paris," she said. This kind of gossip should not be said in the presence of eavesdroppers with, she said, "their ears wagging". She meant the reference to Marxism positively, and, yes, it was true that Miller had been a member of a Maoist group, Gauche prolétarienne, in the 1960s, but for *this* ear-wagging Marxist, a Trotskyist, this was dismaying, defensive talk.

Alienation

There were some Freudian favourite texts in CFAR, discussion of the mirror-stage invariably linked to 'On Narcissism', for example, and lectures often circled around the paper 'A Child is Being Beaten', which would serve for discussion of fantasy and aggression. You could be pretty sure that if dreams were mentioned, then the case of the witty butcher's wife from Chapter 4 of *The Interpretation of Dreams* would be cited and interpreted in line with some dictum from Lacan. They liked Dora as exemplar of hysteria, and, bit by bit, I began to realise that their reference to hysteria was positive rather than pathological. The 'Rat Man case, in contrast, functioned as an illustration of obsessional neurosis, of course. And they especially liked the Wolf Man, a particular fragment of the Wolf Man case, not so much the dream of the white wolves, but the Wolf Man's memory of a hallucination he had had when he was five years old, that he had cut off the tip of his finger. He did not tell his nanny. That might signal castration, fantasy of castration, but, for Lacan, we were reminded many times, this was a hallucinatory experience that he kept to himself, that the Wolf Man as boy had not symbolised. Such refusal of symbolisation might signal a more profound defence, that Lacan called 'foreclosure', a fundamental defence that constituted this patient as a psychotic subject, as one with psychotic structure, psychotic Freudian clinical structure.

They were careful not to point to the hallucination as such as evidence of psychosis. Why? I was intrigued by this, as well as by the debates as to whether this Wolf Man was indeed psychotic or neurotic. This debate, ambiguity as to how the hallucination was functioning for the Wolf Man, pointed to a deep difference between standard psychiatric approaches to hallucinations and Lacan's return to Freud. The *Diagnostic and Statistical Manual of Mental Disorders*, the *DSM* produced by the American Psychiatric Association, specified the hearing of voices as a first-rank symptom of schizophrenia. This psychiatric manual, gathering together a series of symptoms and aggregating them into disease clusters, was in line with the German tradition of psychiatry, a tradition that also underpinned the production of the mental illness categories defined in the ICD, the International Classification of Diseases. The full title of the ICD, which is produced by the World Health Organisation, is the 'International Statistical Classification of Diseases and Related Health Problems'. The 'statistical' aspect of categories of disorder or disease is clearly central to both classification systems, and the aggregation of symptoms is designed to accord with notions of distribution in the general population.

I knew from my work with the Hearing Voices Network in Manchester how poisonous this classification system was. The psychiatrist would be charged with the task of identifying the symptom and determining what contribution it would give to the eventual diagnosis of the patient and then choice of treatment: usually medication, if the patient was lucky, or another more brutal physical treatment such as electroconvulsive therapy, ECT, if they were not. The aim of the treatment was to stop the voices, and the most that could be expected of many other mental health professionals working under the guidance of psychiatrists was that they would find other means of stopping the voices, using, for example, cognitive behavioural therapy, CBT, as a contemporary version of the 'moral treatments' that emerged at the dawn of modern psychiatry in the nineteenth century.

The Lacanian mode of diagnosis was rooted, however, in the French tradition of psychiatry, the tradition in which Lacan himself had been trained. We were told that the French tradition always looked for underlying 'structures', which may manifest themselves in the experience of the individual subject in very different ways, depending on local context and, crucially, on the way the patient accounted for their experience to the psychiatrist. There was an important shift here in the way that psychoanalysis, linked to the German tradition of psychiatry in Freud's own training, conceptualised 'disorder' when it was implanted in the French tradition of psychiatry and was then elaborated by Lacan. Lacan sometimes, it was true, emphasised the 'German' character of Freud's writing, including its psychiatric underpinnings, and this challenged the hostility to things German in chauvinist French psychiatry, but he then reframed Freudian concepts in French psychiatric terms, making use of the contradictions between different French psychiatrists who were his teachers. In some ways this French tradition was much better, for it entailed a shift from observation and mechanical tabulation of symptoms within standardised category systems to a more careful listening to the way that the speech of the patient might indicate something of the underlying structure. Hence the detailed rereading and reinterpretation of what the hallucination of the cut finger might mean in Freud's Wolf Man case history.

On the other hand, this view of distress and of the symptoms that lead someone into analysis was still located in a version of psychiatry, medical psychiatry. Lacan's occasional existentialist take on this – his comment that depression is cowardice, which may be true, for example – did not necessarily completely dislodge psychoanalysis from psychiatry. The psychoanalyst is still in the position of master, the one who will listen and decide what the underlying structure is. A series of sessions on diagnosis were run for the first years by Darian Leader, another initial co-founder of CFAR, and Andrew Hodgkiss, a psychiatrist. We were told that there were three main clinical structures defined by their root in three specific fundamental defence mechanisms defined by Freud: *Verdrängung*, which we translate as 'repression', gave rise to neurotic structure, of which obsessional neurosis was deemed to be a dialect of the most basic hysteria; *Verneinung*, or 'negation', specifically negation of the idea that the mother does not have a phallus, with this denial giving rise to perverse structure and anxiety about the existence, or not, of a powerful Other to which one is beholden; *Verwerfung*, on the other hand, is a more radical defence, which could be translated as rejection but in the Lacanian tradition is a 'foreclosure' in which the key coordinates of the Symbolic order are blanked out completely. Then you have psychosis.

We need, according to Lacan, anchoring points in discourse to prevent the disastrous sliding of concepts under the words we attempt to use to talk about experience. These are signifieds sliding under the signifiers in classical Saussurean terms, and that's the way I described it back in Chapter 3. In more strictly Lacanian terms, and I remember Genie Georgaca putting me right over this, these are signifiers that have dropped to the level of signifieds and then slide under other signifiers. Now you kick away the ladder. Lacan inverts Saussure's image of the signified marked with capital S on top of the bar and the signifier marked with small s below the bar; he inverts it so that the signifier is on top, so it now takes precedence. For Lacan, the signifiers always take precedence over the concepts that seem to be strung along beneath them. What we think we are thinking about is governed by language itself. The anchoring points that operate like the upholstery buttons that hold the fabric and stuffing on a couch in place are, in Lacanian jargon, known as '*points de capiton*'. The 'Name of the Father is just such a *point de capiton* because the Symbolic order is organised around the Law of the Father, the father as necessary mediator of desire, that function that breaks the infant from its potentially all-embracing suffocating relationship with the mother. Castration by the signifier is not a bad thing, but is absolutely necessary. Foreclosure is therefore foreclosure of the Name of the Father, of the signifier of something other than the desire of the mother. What is foreclosed from the Symbolic returns in the Real, Lacan says: that is, what is blanked out from language returns as hallucination.

So, we need to know whether hallucinations are a manifestation of this clinical structure rather than assuming that hallucinations, or the hearing of voices as one instance, are 'symptoms' of psychosis. In some iterations of this story about foreclosure as the basis of psychosis, by Darian Leader, for example, this account was carefully delimited from a psychiatric account. The DSM, Darian liked to say, was printed and sold in edition after edition with ever more categories in it to pay off the mortgage on the American Psychiatric Association's headquarters.

Andrew Hodgkiss, on the other hand, often retreated to psychiatric narratives, warning us that there were different kinds of 'voices': those that accompanied action were fairly benign, while those that directed the patient to carry out certain actions were more likely to be signs of psychosis. Andrew even suggested at one point that while psychosis was, in Lacanian terms, a pathological relationship with the Symbolic order, perhaps it would be possible to treat a genetic predisposition to mental illness as existing in the realm of the Real. Darian sat tactfully silent during such pronouncements, didn't challenge Andrew, as if pretending it hadn't been said. I asked one day how many *points de capiton* were necessary to ensure that there was no psychosis. There was a flurry in the cellar, but no one answered the question. Perhaps they thought I was being facetious, or obsessional.

Separation

There were seminars, the meetings of the particular year groups, which were quite small, not all of us eight turned up to all of them, but small-group work alongside the lectures was also required to be carried out in the 'cartels'. We were required to be in at least two cartels, which would meet at intervals over eighteen months to two years. We needed to gather a cartel together on a topic of our choice ourselves. My two cartels were on the topic of 'discourse', which was a way of exploring a Lacanian take on academic work I was doing, and on 'cartel' itself, that is, reflexively examining the formation of the idea of cartel in the Lacanian school after 1964 and the conception of group that it operated on. A cartel is a small group that can have between three and five people, and so this was a good opportunity to connect with group analysis again.

Erica was in this second cartel, along with Genie Georgaca and Alan Horne, the Gaskell House psychotherapy service manager, who had been one of the key people involved in the Monday morning seminars. This 'cartel cartel' began in December 1998 in Alan's office. This work group – four is the right number, Lacan had said – needed what was called a 'plus one', that is, someone to whom we would be accountable, a figure for whom we would work. This was Hara Pepeli from CFAR. That 'plus one' should notice when the members of the cartel are agreeing with each other too much, and encourage the production of individual outcomes, pieces of work that would be distinct takes on the topic being examined. The idea was that cartels as research groups in the Lacanian school would form and disperse, allowing for a more horizontal network of colleagues than the vertically-organised bureaucratic structures in the IPA. In CFAR we would report on the work in cartels in occasional 'inter-cartel meetings'.

My other cartel, the 'discourse cartel', brought together two trainees in Yorkshire and Dan Heggs, who had returned to Manchester after taking the Kent psychoanalytic studies course and was doing his PhD on origin stories in superhero graphic novels under my supervision. There was some overlap between the two cartels because the question of what the rationale was for cartels involved a conception of discourse, of the structure of discourse that Lacan had explored in his seventeenth seminar. Our plus one was Rik Loose from Dublin.

The four discourses Lacan described in his 1969–1970 seminar – of the university, hysteric, master and analyst – could be seen as a way of analysing the cultural-political context in which psychoanalysis itself developed. The discourse of the university, for example, was a discourse in which all-inclusive knowledge was in the position of agent, knowledge to which all were expected to conform, a version of the adaptation that bureaucratised kinds of psychoanalysis, those kinds promulgated by the IPA, supported. More than that, the different discourses could also, according to some analysts such as Paul Verhaeghe, be used as a diagnostic tool, identifying different structures: obsessional neurosis was replicated and encouraged in the discourse of the university, while hysteria was the domain, as would be expected by the name, of the discourse of the hysteric. The discourse of the master was latently psychotic, and, in a curious twist, often remarked upon in lectures, the discourse of the analyst that provoked a 'hystericisation' of the patient could be seen as perverse.

Everything was pathology. There was no normal. And this, if nothing else, drew attention to the madness of the institution we were part of in our psychoanalytic training. These weren't 'labels' in a strictly psychiatric sense, but I still felt uneasy about reproducing quasi-psychiatric categories in the signifiers 'neurosis', 'psychosis' and 'perversion' that we used to describe social structures. The way they would be used in treatment with our own patients was even more worrying. I would need to face that next.

12

SUPERVISION

Confession and confidentiality

Now I describe the institutional processes that must be navigated in order for the psychoanalyst to find analysands, first patients who might thereby function for training purposes and provide experience of what it is to listen to another person speak. I reflect on what happens in supervision of the practice. Psychotherapy is framed by the institutions in which it operates, and so the versions of Lacan I was working with in different places also had to be tailored to fit. If all the details must be changed, you can never believe what a psychoanalyst says about their patients, and my experience of talking about patients made me wonder if I was betraying more than confidentiality when I did so. Here in this chapter we must talk about truth.

Listening

So, you know this already, I can't tell you exactly what my analysands said because anything they said could be used as clues to their identity. But what I can do is assemble some composite pictures, and I can use the indicators I used in my copious notes on each training case, notes that have now been destroyed. We start with 'A'. A is an academic, and you will begin to see that my patient population is skewed towards those who already know something about psychoanalysis. Before I could find 'A', though, I needed to find a place to do the work.

I was teaching in Bolton Institute at this time, the end of the 1990s, and so I approached the student counselling service of my old place of work in Manchester, MMU, where the head of the service was an old colleague, Carol Lomax, who had moved out of teaching in psychology to practise an avowedly humanist form of therapy. So, you now meet, as did I, a Lacan much more attuned to the existential dimension of being human and struggling with relationships. This Lacan was configured to the demands of the counselling service, though actually this is not such a big distortion of Lacanian practice as you might think. There is an aspect of Lacan's return to Freud that keys into some of the concerns of the more humanistic practitioners of psychoanalysis like Bruno Bettelheim – and Bettelheim's marvellous book *Freud and Man's Soul* had now been published, a book in which he traces through some of the bizarre mistranslations of original German terms in Freud's own writing into the natural-science argot of the 'Standard Edition', edited by James Strachey.

Lacan's own return to Freud is profoundly influenced by Hegel and the phenomenological tradition, and so the implicit link and critical extension of a Rogerian person-centred approach in the MMU counselling service was not so outlandish. The main possible stumbling block was the issue of 'variable length' sessions, but I reassured Carol that this could be a quite minimal variation in the standard fifty-minute 'hour' they followed, a few minutes either way, and, even better, it functioned as a form of interpretation without spelling out the meaning as the analyst saw it. This was music to humanist ears, for the caricature of psychoanalysis that undergraduates had been subjected to had it that the analyst would tell the patient that they were talking to the analyst as if they were their father or mother, say, and then spell out what their dreams really meant. Lacan does not do that, and, like Rogers, he adopts a version of the argument that the 'analysand' or 'person' does at some level in some way know what they want to say. No, not exactly the same, for there is a focus on revealed content in one and *process* of speaking in the other.

The difference between them is that while the Rogerian humanist self-actualising subject is able to make themselves 'congruent', resolve the conflict between who they are and who they have been made to appear to others in order to speak the truth, the Lacanian views this 'barred' or 'divided' subject of the unconscious as always inaccessible, appearing at fleeting moments when the truth of the subject is enunciated, when the 'subject of the enunciation' appears instead of the usual alienated 'subject of the statement'. The subject of the statement is the one who speaks in the tracks of the things that have been said about who they are, and what we might say they have 'internalised' about themselves from those descriptions. I put that term 'internalised' in scare quotes because those statements are still, of course, very much at work on the surface of the language the analysand uses in their everyday life. The subject of the enunciation speaks directly, implicated in what they say, and the analysand may sometimes be shocked when they speak as such, recognising that this is the truth only after they have said it.

Carol agreed to look through her lists of students who had come to the counselling service, and to pass some on to me, on condition that I attended supervision sessions in the service in addition to my own Lacanian supervision. I had a Lacanian supervisor lined up, Michael Kennedy, chosen because he had a background in the object-relations tradition, which was my own first experience of working as a therapist. Michael, who was Chair of CFAR, was an avuncular Australian who would move the location of meetings around London with disarming speed; sometimes we met in a counselling service at the back of Harrods, sometimes at home, once at Marine Ices in Kentish Town, and once in a pub where he downed a pint of beer while I described work with an analysand before he swept away to teach a session down the road at CFAR. I prepared an information sheet about a Lacanian approach and showed it to him; Michael glanced at it and said, "Are you joking?". It wasn't what I had written that was the problem, but that I had assumed that he should see it, seeking reassurance that what I had said was right. I read his response as another indication that humanist and Lacanian approaches could run on parallel tracks. He would listen to me, but he would not guide me when it was clear I already had the competence to work out what to do. It was a first, sharp lesson in a style of supervision that was mainly concerned with overseeing a practice of listening, and listening in such a way as to enable the analysand to speak in such a way that, as Lacan once put it, the unconscious opens.

Supervision in the counselling service focused on what clients might be feeling, while Michael focused on what they were actually saying, tracking the signifiers in their speech. Supervision in the counselling service was concerned with what I was feeling and how I responded to what the client was feeling, aspects of the counselling relationship that sometimes went under the heading of 'counter-transference' in the psychoanalytic tradition. Supervision with Michael, on the other hand, tracked the ways in which my description of what my analysands said sometimes accurately marked the distinctive terms they used and was able to notice that, and the way my description sometimes slipped into general descriptions of what I supposed they were talking about or felt using my own terms.

That assimilation of the analysand's own discourse to my own and the distortions, which then led to a comforting sense that I understood them – in the line of the Imaginary we would say – was the closest we came to conceptualising 'counter-transference'. 'Counter-transference' as such, I knew from Michael's scornful caricatures when he read out extracts of object-relations and Kleinian cases in the CFAR lectures, was too-often treated as some form of telepathy, as if the analyst can magically sense what the analysand is feeling and then process it, turn it into words, and speak an accurate description back in the form of an interpretation.

Just as I started to see students in the MMU counselling service at the end of 1999, there was a problem. I got an academic post back at MMU, and this would probably make it difficult for students in the psychology department to access the counselling service as a confidential secure space. If students as clients saw me wandering around the service, their own sense of confidentiality would be thrown into question. I contacted the counselling service of the University of Manchester across the road through a friend and political contact who was working there, Rachel Pollard, and there were other people I had bumped into in critical psychology meetings. Now, three weeks after I had begun working in a humanistic environment, I had to pitch Lacan to a meeting of the counselling team that included practitioners of cognitive analytic therapy, CAT. A new introductory outline was called for, and a slightly different Lacan.

He could be more psychoanalytic now, of course, but also needed to orient more explicitly to patterns in discourse. The University of Manchester counselling service group, led by Steve Potter, wanted to know more about diagnosis, about how I might determine whether someone might be able to engage with the therapeutic process or whether they might be too fragile, the closest we, together in the group, got to indications of psychotic structure. The advantage was that they would be willing to circulate a notice to staff in the university, and so I would not see undergraduate students and my analysands would know that this approach was Lacanian. I had supervision on Wednesday mornings with Gill Barnett in the service, during which I tried to explain in more detail what I was doing in the sessions, which was useful. We set things up, and so Mondays then became a hectic full day in which I continued to see MMU 'peeps' – my very non-analytic term for my clients, persons, patients, analysands – while winding down work with that service, also saw Manchester University peeps, and then drove down to Chester for my own analytic sessions; now Ian, Amelia's peep.

Speaking

I had to listen to them and I had to speak about them. To be honest, I felt bad speaking about them. Supervision was fine, and the very different kinds of supervision I experienced were spaces for thinking while speaking about what I had heard, much more so than scribbling notes and then staring at them. Well, that's what you would expect in a Lacanian frame: writing is in the realm of statements, empirical description, which is necessarily alienated from experience, shut out by the wall of written language in a quite explicit way, while speaking allows surprising connections between signifiers to appear unbeknownst to you in an enunciation of the truth of the encounter or, at least, a little closer to it. Encourage psychotics to write, we were told, rather than unravel their speech.

Case presentations were another matter, a perfect occasion for concealment rather than truth, for the fabrication of a narrative rather than the puzzling over things said that do not make sense. Nevertheless, I agreed to do a case presentation at a Saturday Freudian Field seminar in London, that is, a joint meeting between CFAR and the Millerian group, the London Circle, a separate group that CFAR was still keen to be aligned with. As a CFAR trainee I was anxious I might be trashed as an object lesson. The discussant was a prominent Millerian brought over from Paris, Marie-Hélène Brousse. I wanted to talk about the way that the institutions we work in frame the kind of work we do, which in the case of the analysand I described, was an obsessional academic who wanted things kept to time, and who marvelled at my ability to judge the length of sessions without looking at my watch. (There was a clock on the filing cabinet out of her sight.) The question was not only what kind of object the analysand is turned into in the bureaucratic systems of a counselling service, but also what kind of object we are turned into as analysts, as objects of surveillance in different regulatory systems that are supposed to guarantee that the service is an ethical service.

Richard Klein was there at the Freudian Field seminar, he was now one of the kingpins of the London Millerians, after leaving CFAR, and I could see Bernard Burgoyne from CFAR, at the back of the room, by turns worried and relieved, chuckling when I finished my talk and Marie-Hélène Brousse delivered her verdict. She said that the task of the psychoanalyst is to position themselves as *objet petit a*, as object of love, as loveable. I said that I had tried very hard to present myself as loveable, and she laughed, phew, everyone laughed, and she said I had spoken the truth about my encounter. I was happy with this, but puzzled about what 'truth' it was that really was at stake here.

On the train home I wondered if I would be able to refuse to do clinical case presentations in the future. The 'truth' that was present there could only, even if the speaker was very canny, be the truth of the psychoanalyst. We didn't know when things changed for the analysand in the sessions, and it was, after all, a fundamental precept of Lacanian psychoanalysis that the truth of the subject in the process of enunciation was as something realised by the analysand, the one who was speaking, and may only be realised by them after the event, *Nachträglich*.

Michael Kennedy once lent me a copy of Marie Cardinal's book *The Words to Say It*, originally published in the mid-1970s, in which she describes her own analysis; she knows something has changed at the end of the analysis, but not what it was, neither does she ever arrive at an accurate representation of what the problem was. Michael was telling me not to be so sure that I knew exactly what was going on the minds of my analysands. The case presentations I heard, and the one I had just presented, were just too neat and tidy to accurately represent what actually went on in the sessions. I was sure that my analysand would not recognise in the truth that had been valued at the end of the talk by Marie-Hélène Brousse anything like their own truth, the truth of the subject who had spoken to me in the closed clinical space. I felt a fraud. Well, that's not unusual, but I also felt that I had colluded in a particular kind of institutional practice. It was all very well talking about the way that clinical institutions framed analysis, but we needed to think about how the institution of the clinical case presentation itself also reframed what went on and misled those who listened to these untrue psychoanalytic tales.

Joining

I could not yet join CFAR – I had to complete the training first – but I could join the local Millerian group that had by now mutated from being the London Circle into being the London Society of the New Lacanian School, the LSNLS. It now organised completely separately from CFAR, announcing that 'the Freudian Field has accomplished its task in the UK'. Darian Leader complained that the NLS were treating CFAR people simply as 'human resources', and objected to 'fanciful new terminology and dogmatic statements' in the Millerian groups, giving a link to a book by Colette Soler and followers while cautioning that it also contained 'rhetoric which is just as dodgy as that of their opponents'. Frying pans and fires, the internal battles were hotting up. I asked Heather Menzies, now Chamberlain, by email how I could join the London Society of the NLS. She told me I should contact the people she had suggested in the emails she had already given me. I tracked back through my emails to check. Nothing. I asked again, and got a sharp reply that she had already told me. She wore her hair ravelled up high with grey streaks shooting up the sides, and I had images of one of the mad queens from *Alice through the Looking Glass*. This encounter was either out of Lewis Carroll or Franz Kafka, perhaps a combination of the two. I eventually had two interviews in 2001 to join, one with Roger Litten and one with Bogdan Wolf.

The one with Roger was on the morning of a meeting at the Tavistock Clinic of the 'Diagonal', one of the many Millerian front organisations that sprouted up and then disappeared. To be at the Tavistock is a sign that you have arrived at the dead centre of British psychoanalysis. The Diagonal, a 'Conversation in the Diagonal' publication from 2000 announced, was designed to build an 'English-speaking working community in Europe' and it included analysts from Denmark, Israel, Poland, Belgium, the UK and France. That Saturday in May 2001 the Millerians hired the top floor of the clinic, and the first few speakers seemed to treat this as an occupation of an IPA stronghold, a victory. Jean-Pierre Klotz from Bordeaux gloated in his introduction to the day, looking around the room, and repeating the words with some jealous admiration to mark that we were here: "The Tavistock!" They were going to bring it alive.

Roger Litten had turned up for my LSNLS interview with dark glasses, which he kept on during the course of the encounter. "The question," he said, "is not what we can do for you but," and I could easily predict what would come next after the meaningful pause, "what you can do for us." I reminded him that I had given papers at LSNLS events and would be speaking there that afternoon. "Yes," he said, "well, you could think of your application as being like the case of K in Kafka's *Trial* before the door of the Law." I was puzzled. "You may discover that the door was meant for you, and was already open." "O … K," I said slowly, and then Roger reminded me that two interviews were necessary and that then the LSNLS committee would decide.

At the other interview with Bogdan in a café in Camden, I was told that although I was currently training with CFAR, and there was no reason why I should not be a member of both organisations. "At some future point," Bogdan said, "You might need to make a choice." He told me, after I talked about travelling from Manchester to London for meetings, including LSNLS meetings that were not part of the CFAR training, that at one point he had lived in Newcastle, much further from London, and that, "well, you have to pay with your body". I agreed, and then Bogdan asked me about my interest in Marxism, concluding the interview with the observation that it would be interesting to hear more about Marxism, about "your Marxism", he said, in the LSNLS. They let me in, and then I had to really pay, pay an annual subscription.

Five years into my training I was beginning to ease off attending the Saturday lectures. The travel from Manchester to London was an ordeal by that time, with 'improvements' to the line at weekends leading to delays of two or three hours. Sometimes I could not get to London at all, and needed to turn back at a station en route where rail replacement buses were picking up passengers.

When I talked to Lindsay my tutor and Michael my supervisor about applying for membership of CFAR, they talked to the Training Committee, and the mysterious process bringing this process to an end started to become more complicated. Requirements for training were ratcheted up, I felt, and it was unclear whether this was really, as I was advised when a response was relayed to me, because CFAR needed to comply with UKCP. I knew that these last phases of training in CFAR often unleashed paranoid speculation among trainees about what the Training Committee really wanted, and I still had buzzing Bernard Burgoyne's reassuring words to Jacques-Alain Miller in the CFAR bulletin that training might take around ten years, as well as suspicions on the part of other trainees that somehow they were writing for the wrong big Other.

I was also, of course, six years into analysis with Amelia, who had to listen to my whining about wanting to finish the training. She didn't seem impressed. Well, I couldn't see her, so I couldn't be sure, but I guessed that she thought I was complaining about nothing, that I had it easy. That's transference. She knew well that I had taken time off to travel for work during these years, but I couldn't so easily conceal from her that some of that time had been spent travelling for pleasure. The spring term in 2002, for example, had been completely wiped out, and I'd had to write to the Training Committee to explain my absence from lectures, and to reassure them that I had made back-up arrangements with my analysands, and given contact information for other analysts that they could contact if need be while I was away. It was risky to leave them for three months, with a real danger that they would decide not to return to me when I returned to Manchester.

At least Amelia didn't report to the Training Committee on my progress. By now I had upped my sessions with her from two to three times a week. The IPA were making a big deal about one of the key planks of a psychoanalytic training being five-times-a-week personal analysis, and CFAR were under pressure on this. This increased the cost of analysis by fifty per cent, of course, but fortunately I could have these three sessions on the same day with breaks between to ponder over why Amelia had cut it at twenty minutes, or fifteen, or sometimes less. Maybe she was sick of me whining too.

My tutor Lindsay looked at drafts of the four papers I wanted to submit to the Training Committee, and made me think about who I was writing for, or, rather, what persona I was assuming as I wrote. This is what I understood by her cryptic comment that I should reflect on what 'semblant' was at work in the writing. This threw me into an anxious search, after I left that tutorial, for an explanation. The term 'semblant' could have been linked to the signifier 'imaginarise' that was appearing in CFAR discourse at that moment, referring to a discursive production that was neither claiming to be directly expressing something of the Real, which would anyway be impossible, nor following the tracks of the Symbolic, locating itself in current shared ways of describing the world, which could anyway be viewed as conformism, but was of the Imaginary; that is, imagining, in this case, transparent communication of meaning from author to reader. To 'imaginarise', then, would be to turn something into an imaginary production that neither attended to its symbolic construction nor to the Real. What Lindsay might have meant was that my writing was phoney, was something artificial for an audience. But my four papers clearly needed to be for a particular audience, so I felt trapped and more anxious.

Michael warned me that the Training Committee expected that I should have experience of working with more than one supervisor on the training, a requirement that had not cropped up before, and so I quickly arranged another supervisor, Patricia Touton-Victor, a French Millerian. That certainly was a different experience, and was very useful. She posed questions about my practice that Michael and I had taken for granted, 'imaginarised' together you might say. In one session, for example, Patricia asked me why I had reported a dream by an analysand and had not painstakingly picked through different elements of the dream with them. It wasn't that I was being lazy, and she wasn't accusing me of that. But she pointedly reminded me that dreams are not free-standing vignettes that express the preoccupations of the analysand at a particular point in their lives. No, she said, they are rather like wells tapping into something of their unconscious lives.

By 2003 I was travelling down to London, there and back in one day on occasion, managing to fit in supervision with Patricia, a tutorial with Lindsay, and then two supervision sessions with Michael. Lindsay eventually gave the go-ahead and so I submitted my papers to the Training Committee at the end of May, saying in a covering letter that I had now seen eleven analysands, most of them for over eight months and at least two of them for over two years, the two that I wrote about. Silence. Things were not to be straightforward. I had a message some months later from the Training Committee that they would like to meet with me to discuss my clinical practice. It wasn't until the beginning of November that I met Astrid Gessert and Vincent Dachy, two members of the Training Committee, at Vincent's apartment in central London, after I had a supervision meeting with Michael where I wondered aloud about how the meeting might go. "Just tell them about the work you are doing," Michael said. At the apartment, Vincent said, "We have read the theory papers, and," a pause, "no comment."

These were two papers I had also worked on as journal articles. One was called 'Jacques Lacan, barred psychologist', and was on the way that Lacanian psychoanalysis was the antithetical opposite of psychology. The other was an explication and review of a three-way dialogue between Ernesto Laclau, Slavoj Žižek, and the feminist queer theorist, Judith Butler. I was not sure whether this 'no comment' meant they liked the papers well enough and would accept them, or not. "What we wanted to know more about," Astrid said, "is something we could not really get from your two clinical papers, that is, what your own practice is like." I struggled to answer, speaking about the place where I saw my analysands, and how I might speak a little too much in some of the sessions, and, a bit defensive this, how I might sometimes over-intellectualise in the description of the cases, but this was after the event, an attempt to make sense of what had happened. I was not at all as sure in the sessions as it might appear from reading the cases. We went around this a few times, and then, in less than an hour, Vincent called time, and I left, unsure what the outcome would be, whether there would be some next steps, or what.

A letter from Darian Leader for the Training Committee dated 4 December 2003 was carefully balanced between two paragraphs. The first paragraph said that my theoretical papers and 'academic writing skills', as he put it, 'managed to upstage the clarity of your input to the direction of the treatment in the clinical papers'. My heart sank at the suggestion that followed this, that the Committee thought I should have more clinical experience and would 'strongly recommend' a placement in a 'psychiatric setting' and more supervision. 'However', the second paragraph began, 'we do not think that the discrepancy between your theoretical and clinical papers was a reason not to grant you membership of CFAR'. Is this yes or no, I thought. The letter suggested that I might myself think it would be a good idea to gain more clinical experience, but that they would let me decide. This was not an 'additional requirement', and they would welcome me into membership of CFAR, they said, 'at the moment that you choose'.

If you think that six-and-a-half years of psychoanalysis had made me less impatient, then think again. I did hesitate, oscillated between being a compliant trainee who had fully internalised the idea that I was not yet ready, and one who wanted to get this over and done with. I had a lingering unfounded suspicion that the rules might change if I did not act fast. So I did. A few days later I wrote back saying that 'I feel that the best conditions for me to take forward my work will be in the context of CFAR'. And that was that. Almost. A letter at the beginning of February the following year, 2004, from Michael Kennedy as Chair of CFAR welcomed me as a new member. I remembered that when Lacan had been given membership of the Société Parisienne de Psychanalyse in the early 1930s he had promised to continue his personal analysis with Rudolf Loewenstein, one of the three founders, with Heinz Hartmann and Ernst Kris, of the US-American current of 'ego psychology'. Lacan immediately broke his promise.

I had not promised to carry on my analysis with Amelia, and in fact I ended my analysis with her just before the letter offering that I make a choice over membership of CFAR arrived. It was a risky move, a leap into the unknown. I do not know what she thought about this. Many possible ideas about that, about what she thought, what I supposed her to know, occurred to me, however now it was time to let go and move on. But I paid for it, something horribly superegoic in me told me that I would enjoy representing CFAR at United Kingdom Council for Psychotherapy meetings for a few years. They asked me to do it. I agreed. By May 2004 I was at my first 'Psychoanalytic and Psychodynamic Section' meeting of the UKCP at the Guild of Psychotherapists in Nelson Square. It was an opportunity to get to know colleagues who became friends in other training organisations, a time during which I got tangled up with psychoanalytic resistance to state regulation. I had overcome my own resistance to psychoanalysis, but not completely, and though I was sold on the practice, I was not convinced by the rather paranoiac attempts by adepts to find Freud everywhere. The next four chapters focus on the problematic assumption that what goes on between two people in the strange space of the consulting room can be extrapolated to what goes on in the outside world, around the world.

13

ENLIGHTENMENT

Second nature in Brazil

We turn now to the temptation that besets almost every psychoanalyst after their training, those for whom psychoanalysis has turned into a world view, to 'apply' it here, there and everywhere. These next four chapters look at attempts to contextualise and apply psychoanalysis, beginning with Brazil as one country that has taken a different path through to modernity, with different competing conceptions of the relationship between culture and nature. You will encounter many competing schools of psychoanalysis, glued together by the narcissism of minor differences. This application of psychoanalysis also begins in the very process of questioning it, looking for something different from Western preconceptions in another strange dialectic of Enlightenment.

Culture

Erica met him in the elevator during the 1999 biennial congress of the SIP, the Sociedad Interamericana de Psicología, in Caracas, Venezuela. He was a tall, slim man with short, dark hair, a Brazilian psychoanalyst who had just attended her talk on developmental psychology and deconstruction. Christian Ingo Lenz Dunker, Chris, went back to his hotel room to tell his wife, Ana-Cris, "I've met the woman of my life." I was in bed for most of the congress with food poisoning, images of the crab dish I had eaten in someone's informal, economy house-restaurant during our visit to Cuba swimming through my head.

Cuba was the location for extraordinary biennial discussions about psychoanalysis from 1987 onwards, the site that year of the SIP congress, to the mid-1990s, with Lacanians and other analysts invited to Havana by Fernando González Rey, who was, at one point, vice-rector of the university, and Albertina Mitjáns Martínez, his successor. González Rey, who had studied for his PhD in 'activity theory' in Moscow, had closely followed the discussions about the re-emergence of psychoanalysis in the

Soviet Union. He had later relocated to Brazil with Mitjáns Martínez, where their critical work on subjectivity included discussion of the links between those two theoretical traditions. Psychoanalysis was alive and well in Latin America.

In Brazil it was thriving, as Chris Dunker explained when he visited Manchester in 2000, with a concentration of psychoanalysts in the main cities, almost on a par with Argentina to the south, a country that had supplied wave after wave of analysts to the rest of Latin America, particularly during the mass emigration of radicals during the military dictatorship and 'dirty war' from 1974 to 1983. The years of dictatorship had seen a curious double-process of emigration and occupation in which a generation of radical psychoanalysts had fled, and in which a new generation of less radical psychoanalysts had moved in to occupy the empty institutional positions. Some psychoanalysts claim that you need democracy for clinical work to flourish, but actually psychoanalysis has survived under some quite authoritarian regimes, whether that was Hungary between the two world wars or South Africa under apartheid; the question for the regime is whether what goes on in the clinic is confined to psychologising social issues, in which case there is no problem, or whether it might also involve politicising analysands.

Marxists like the Kleinian psychoanalyst Marie Langer had to leave. After a life facing fascism, moving from Nazi Vienna to Spain to fight with the republicans against Franco in the 1930s, Marie Langer had settled in Buenos Aires to build a psychoanalytic practice there. One day in the clinic one of her analysands warned her that she was on a paramilitary death list. She interpreted this as a manifestation of transference, which, for Kleinians, would also necessarily be a manifestation of aggressive, unconscious fantasies about the destruction of parental figures. That night she packed up and left, travelling north, spending time in Nicaragua to work as a child psychoanalyst with the Sandinistas in the 1980s. As a Kleinian, she was, of course, a key figure, an iconic example of what could be done to link Marxism and psychoanalysis, a link promoted by Bob Young and some colleagues in the *Free Associations* journal project in the UK.

So, many psychoanalysts, including Kleinians and radical Lacanians like Néstor Braunstein had to leave. Psychoanalysis in a private space in which the analysand could talk freely was itself viewed as a threat to the dictatorship, just as the practice had been viewed by many other totalitarian regimes. In Argentina there was also an antisemitic aspect to the regime, with psychoanalysis and the left assumed to be part of a conspiracy managed by the Jews as puppetmasters, which posed a particular threat to analysts like Langer and Braunstein. There was another unpleasant side to the process: the disappearance of so many Kleinians and other IPA psychoanalysts from Argentina opened up opportunities for more Lacanians to move in. This is not to say that Lacanians are to the right of Kleinians; one could argue, against many of those involved in *Free Associations* journal, that the reverse is the case. It is impossible to settle the matter one way or another. However, in this specific context, Lacanians became the dominant psychoanalytic current in Argentina. They were viewed as arrogant, and a joke I heard told at different times across Latin America expresses some stereotyped suspicion of them, that the superego is like having a drunken Argentinian inside your head. I have never seen Amelia drunk.

Back to Brazil, and a no less unwholesome history for psychoanalysis, with unresolved disputes about the role analysts played in the course of the resistance and in the pay of the military regime there, a regime that had already seized power in 1964 and that lasted until 1985. On the one hand, there was much interest in psychoanalysis during those years among the left, and some of the most well-known cultural-political figures in the resistance, like Augusto Boal who developed a theatre of the oppressed in poor communities, went into exile. Boal went into Lacanian psychoanalysis when he was in France. On the other hand, some IPA psychoanalysts who worked for the regime, including directly for the military, were implicated in torture. Many psychoanalysts were able to maintain a strict divide between the public realm and the private space of the clinic, listening to horror stories of torture and resistance from their analysands while staying neutral about politics, at the very least refraining from speaking out. It was said that, just as nineteenth-century European bourgeois families would equip the older sons for business and send the younger ones into the Church, so in Brazil the younger sons were sent to train as psychoanalysts.

Chris Dunker brought this history of an alternative path to modernity, bloodier and with a complicated relationship to the formation of subjectivity, to Manchester when he came to us for postdoctoral study visits supervised primarily by Erica, and for journeys to London with me to see what Lacanian psychoanalysis was like in Britain. An email from Chris after his first visit in 2000 was a nice reminder of how intensely psychoanalytic our discussions had been. We had given Chris a Santa Claus doll to take home for his son Mathias, and Chris said it was, for Mathias, a kind of metonymic representation of his father's travel to England: 'He said "Linguaterra" for it, that means "Language + Land", very properly an interpretation for his father's desire.' The questions Chris raised were not only about our much more cautious approach to politics but also about the way that psychoanalysis in other parts of the world conceptualised the relationship between psychoanalysis and other kinds of cures in quite novel ways; what it was to be eclectic in psychotherapy took on a whole different meaning.

The narrative spun by the Frankfurt School for the development of psychoanalysis in Europe, and swallowed wholesale by *Free Associations* to orient radicals to the IPA in Britain as if it were a left-of-centre democratic force, was that the kind of repression entailed by civilisation reconfigured the relationship between culture and nature. Adorno and Horkheimer's book *Dialectic of Enlightenment*, for example, includes description and interpretation of the figure of Odysseus on his ship. Odysseus orders his crew to plug their ears with wax so they cannot hear the Sirens, and to bind him to the mast so he can still direct the ship without being able to fall prey to their deadly alluring calls that would draw them all to death on the rocks. Odysseus, Adorno and Horkheimer argue, is emblematic of the modern ego, beset by temptation, by unconscious desire, and tied to order in order to survive.

Our Western 'Enlightenment', then, promotes a peculiar form of reason as the centrepiece of culture that is set against nature viewed as something dangerous, out of control. That form of reason, as Michel Foucault was to show in his reworking of these themes in his analysis of the development of modernity, thoroughly individualised human experience, with the collective also viewed as dangerous, as mob rule, closer to nature. We pay the price for our reason with apparatuses of surveillance and confession. It is difficult, one of the leading writers in the second generation of the Frankfurt School, Jürgen Habermas, pointed out, to see much of a 'dialectic' in Adorno and Horkheimer's historical analysis of Enlightenment, but he also scorned attempts to find forms of resistance in what Foucault called 'the body and its pleasures', seeing in that an appeal to unreason, something that could itself issue in something very like fascism. Habermas shifted attention to the role of language in a kind of parallel track to Lacan's return to Freud; and the third generation of the Frankfurt School, particularly Axel Honneth, then picked up Hegel's account of the master-slave dialectic to retrieve from it a psychoanalytic account of child development that emphasised 'recognition', a quasi-Rogerian account in which Honneth often seemed to forget the role of language in the talking cure altogether.

Psychoanalysis, for most of the writers in the first generation of the Frankfurt School, steered a course between outright endorsement of contemporary culture on the one hand and calls for a return to nature on the other. Contemporary society was moulded by the culture industries, which peddled images of satisfaction and freedom that were downright hypocritical, luring the customer to buy more and more in the futile hope that they would be satisfied, and inviting them to believe that they were all the more free in doing so. Such isolated, self-contained individual freedom of choice is exactly one of the tropes of modern subjectivity that Slavoj Žižek, who started his career working on the Frankfurt School, named 'the sublime object of ideology'.

Appeals to nature were, for the Frankfurt School, part of the problem, for every image of nature that is sold to us has the effect of distancing ourselves all the more from nature as such. Instead, psychoanalysis was a practice of critical reflection on what had become our 'second nature', the deep sense that we were separate individuals, men or women with particular kinds of normative heterosexual needs that needed to be satisfied, as if nature was what drove us and culture was what held us back. This term 'second nature' was fruitfully used in accounts of culture and ideology by the Hungarian Marxist Georg Lukács; and then by the US-based socialist feminist Donna Haraway, and picked up by Bob Young, her publisher in the UK, for critiques of scientific reason and for a radical, Kleinian reading of Freud. One could say that one aspect of the 'dialectic' of Enlightenment was that we were also at the very same time subject to an ideological framing of culture as being the only thing that saved us and improved us; we were necessarily set against a nature that would otherwise chain us to repetitive barbaric behaviour.

But in Brazil, Chris Dunker claimed, things were quite otherwise. While Western European psychoanalysts still subscribed to a version of the ethic of 'abstinence' that Freud recommended during the treatment, Brazilian psychoanalysts had to reckon with their analysands combining their analytic treatment with a range of other cures. Freud wanted his analysands to abstain from new sexual experiences during the treatment, for those experiences would thereby, he reasoned, muddle things in the consulting room, confusing what was happening during the talking cure with what was happening in the real world, in other practices that went direct to the body. Chris Dunker's analysands, however, would go one day to an afro-Brazilian Candomblé ritual, and turn up the next to psychoanalysis. We knew from Erica's PhD student, Ilana Mountian, that drug practices in Brazil had a mixed 'hybrid' relationship with standard clinical treatments, with the ingestion of substances during Santo Daime worship operating as adjacent to rather than in opposition to psychoanalysis. Chris argued that Brazilian 'second nature' was embedded in contradictory forms of life that needed to be comprehended as cultural syncretism. Psychoanalysis was powerful in Brazil, but it was not the only game in town. It could not be.

Nature

Chris Dunker emphasised the importance of culture in psychoanalysis, but this belied quite deep assumptions about human nature in Brazilian psychoanalysis, particularly around questions of gender. Chris insisted that there was no feminist debate in Brazil, a claim that corresponded with what Erica's student Ilana was telling her at the time, but we, Erica and I, were sure that this was more a reflection of the framing of cultural issues by psychoanalytic discourse than an accurate reflection of what was actually going on in political movements. "Ilana is using Heidegger to do the same kind of work as debates in artificial intelligence did for me," Erica argued; feminist arguments as such would come later for her. During our first visit to Brazil in 2002 to speak at various psychoanalytic meetings organised by Chris, we encountered Brazilian feminist Lacanians, such as Ana Laura Prates Pacheco, who were beginning to work with the ideas of queer theorist Judith Butler, but these were only first indications that distinctions between supposedly 'natural' and determinedly 'cultural' aspects of gender were being taken up from Freud's own writings and worked through.

These distinctions were second nature to us, taking for granted the argument that Juliet Mitchell made in her 1974 book *Psychoanalysis and Feminism* where she pointed to one of the key footnotes in Freud's 1905 text 'Three Essays on the Theory of Sexuality'. In this footnote, Freud argued that the common-sensical opposition between 'masculine' and 'feminine' confused three different meanings: sometimes the terms were used as equivalent to biological difference, sometimes as equivalent to sociological distinctions, and sometimes to refer to the difference between activity and passivity. Freud himself wanted to stay with the third opposition, between activity and passivity, and viewed the libido as being 'masculine', a problematic and ideological assumption. But at the same time he was usefully opening up a distinction in psychoanalysis between the level of biological discourse in which we refer to 'male' and 'female', cultural discourse in which we refer to 'boys' and 'girls', and sexual identity in which we refer to 'masculinity' and 'femininity'. These three sets of oppositional terms have quite different consequences for how we understand subjectivity, and we needed to take these distinctions seriously, Mitchell argued, if we were also to understand the difference between description and prescription in psychoanalysis; she writes on the first page of her introduction to that book that 'psychoanalysis is not a recommendation *for* a patriarchal society, but an analysis *of* one'.

When the Brazilian analysts we met talked about feminism they were also, at the same time, talking about femininity in just the way that Freud continued to do in many of his writings, and that Lacan continued to do in many of his seminars. The formulae of 'sexuation' that Lacan sketched out in his 1972–1973 Seminar XX didn't help; those formulae could have been a good way of distinguishing between the side of the 'man' and the side of the 'woman' as ideological constructs on the one hand, and masculinity and femininity on the other. Most of the time, and certainly most often in Brazilian Lacanian psychoanalysis, it seemed as if the side of woman was site of a no less ideological picture of femininity and hysterical protest. In other words, this version of feminism simply switched the value given to masculinity and femininity, to value women's sexuality as 'other' and problematise men's as 'phallic'. This gave a peculiar valence to the hystericisation of the analysand in the clinic, making it equivalent to feminising them, a semiotic provocation that is sometimes also found in French Lacanian debate. In place of the derogation of femininity and hysteria in much popular discourse, most Lacanians here, at least, were idealising femininity; this was a repetition of the motif of 'convulsive beauty' that Lacan himself had idealised when he flirted with Surrealism in the early 1930s. Nature was still in command.

Ana Laura Prates Pacheco, who we met in São Paulo at Chris Dunker's house to talk about these issues, was in the advance guard of a Lacanian feminist return to Freud, and was beginning to open up these distinctions again. Ana Laura was also a member of the School of Psychoanalysis of the Forums of the Lacanian Field, that is, followers of Colette Soler who had broken from Jacques-Alain Miller at the Barcelona congress in 1998, or been expelled, depending on who you talked to. The Solerian second 'international' had been formed in December 2001, and claimed to have really effectively begun with the dissolution of Lacan's own school back in 1980, the year before Lacan died, the year before Miller took the reins at the head of the École de la cause freudienne and then the World Association of Psychoanalysis, which we knew in Britain as the WAP. This was a retroactive reading of events if ever there was one.

Ana Laura was happy to talk to me, but still worried that I was a member of Miller's group in London, even when I explained that there was a large overlap of members with CFAR, and that the Millerians were not yet powerful enough to demand obedient undivided loyalty. Some people see Lacan as the L. Ron Hubbard of the psychoanalytic movement – they treat his work as religion masquerading as science – some see that as a positive comparison, and some view Jacques-Alain Miller as David Miscavige, the new ecclesiastical leader. The Reformation-style splits in Scientology are indeed mirrored across many different organisations. The split between the Millerians and Solerians had been very bitter in Brazil, with the matter still not resolved even if, or perhaps because of the existence of rival schools affiliated to rival international organisations. It did look as if the split was more a power play between two individuals and then two separate institutions than down to serious doctrinal differences. There were two possible dividing lines that became magnified in importance to justify the separation of the two Lacanian traditions. One was over sexuality, with the Solerians being much more forthright over their support for different sexual orientations, an issue that was of burning importance in debates in France over the legitimacy of so-called 'gay marriage', a question on which many of the Millerians were then still equivocal, hedging their bets until there was a clear pronouncement by Miller. On this question Soler and the Solerians could be seen as being more open to feminism, more to the 'left' if you like, and this was important to the context in which Ana Laura was writing.

The other issue concerned the ideal form of organisation of a Lacanian School. After 1998 Miller spoke often about the importance of 'the School', and his followers parroted this line, understanding by it that it meant active and loyal participation in it as a condition for being a psychoanalyst. Lacan's dictum that 'the psychoanalyst derives his authorisation only from himself', a phrase that appears in his 'Proposition of 9 October 1967 on the Psychoanalyst of the School' was worried over and, much in the manner of reading a Biblical text, reinterpreted to mean that such 'authorisation' must be in the context of the School.

The Solerians claimed that just as the IPA had become bureaucratised and dogmatic, so the Millerian School had become hierarchical and manipulative. They accused Miller of distorting another aspect of the 1967 'Proposition', which was the institution of 'the pass'; an institutional device for determining who could become a member of the School. In 'the pass', the candidate gives testimony of their analysis to two 'passers', and these passers take that testimony, as they understand it, to a cartel, four people who make up the panel that decides on the basis of what they hear whether the candidate should be given membership. This testimony of personal analysis during training became extended to function as a higher-grade ritual to which analysts should subject themselves to show their loyalty, to work their way up the quasi-Masonic apparatus of the School. Millerians then marked themselves out not by specific theoretical innovations, according to followers of Soler, Solerians downplaying how Miller's own emphasis on 'the Real' did indeed become a signature motif, a sign of allegiance in some presentations by his acolytes. There are changes of perspective and different competing orientations in Miller's innovative work, a healthy contradictoriness that is sometimes overshadowed by the elaboration of a distinctive period of work that the Millerians came to call 'the later Lacan', the Lacan of the Real and the sinthome. Rather, they indicate who they are most loyal to by using phrases such as 'as Miller has noted' when referring to phrases in Lacan's seminars. This was caricatured by the São Paulo Solerians during the worst phase of the split, when they would say to each other in the morning, "Good morning," a pause, "as Jacques-Alain Miller would say."

We attended a celebration party after a successful PhD thesis defence, held in an expensive apartment overlooking Avenida Paulista that belonged to a friend of Chris and Ana Laura. The student was, we were told, a Solerian, but we were then warned that there would be some Millerians there. They were pointed out to us – "and those two" sitting on the couch next to the Solerian, "they are Melmanians". What, what were they? They didn't have different shaped bits of rubber on their foreheads to easily distinguish them from others, as rival species from different planets would do in *Star Trek*. The plot thickened. I had heard murmurings about a 'Forums' group in CFAR sympathetic to Soler, but there weren't, as far as I knew, any 'Melmanians' in London. It turned out that there was a third 'international' on the Lacanian scene.

Charles Melman, a psychiatrist, was co-founder of a network called the Association Lacanienne Internationale. When Jacques-Alain Miller began to work with his future father-in-law, Lacan, it quickly became apparent that he would need to undergo analysis himself in order to become a member of the school, a precondition, of course, for taking over as leader when the dad died. Miller went into analysis with Melman, and something of the transference, perhaps what we discussed in CFAR as a 'negative therapeutic reaction' lingered on, and worse, something negative in the desire of the analyst, Melman, who spoke about the analysis. He should not have done so, of course. Melman's signature dish is the 'real father', and this plays its way out in some more obviously reactionary pronouncements in Paris against gay marriage, in the argument that to enter the Symbolic order one must have a real father and mother. Otherwise, again, Freud's phrase 'narcissism of minor differences' did seem apposite here to make sense of these rivalries.

Assemblages

We are still in 2002 here for the moment, still early days in some of the fractures in the Lacanian psychoanalytic movement. Chris Dunker took us to different seminars at universities in São Paulo, another lesson in the diversity of the theoretical approach in Brazilian psychoanalysis, way beyond the differences between the Millerians, Solerians and Melmanians. We were given the titles of the seminars we would run, and when we balked at, say 'Adorno and psychoanalysis', saying we knew little about that, Chris would cheerfully reassure us, saying that there was going to be an 'Adornian' there who would do most of the talking. There were journals devoted to different combinations of theory, including one exploring connections between Winnicott and Heidegger. We were warned that the hard-line Kleinians really did interpret the transference and would use psychoanalytic theory to interpret the underlying reasons why people objected to them. A story circulated of an analysand who went to a new Kleinian psychoanalyst in São Paulo, and at the beginning of the first session they took a drink from the water fountain in the corner of the consulting room. After the analysand had sat down again, the psychoanalyst said, "When you have finished sucking my dick you can tell me why you have come for analysis."

When we had finished our work, Chris Dunker gave us the choice between going up to Rio for Carnival or going down to Porto Alegre for the second World Social Forum, a leftist political gathering of the alter-globalisation movement. The deciding factor was that Chris had been brought up in Porto Alegre, gone to school there, and had not been back since. We flew down south, hired a car, and looked up his old haunts before going to the World Social Forum. Chris talked often about 'coolture'. It's easy to mock. Our Portuguese is almost non-existent, filtered through bad Spanish, and Chris was an ebullient translator, day after day navigating everyday discourse and theoretical debates. It was exhausting enough for us. Our late call on Porto Alegre meant that hotels were practically full up with visiting activists from around the world. We managed to find one triple bedroom, and we two listened to Chris snore loudly through the night, sometimes talking in his sleep, on at least one occasion shouting out, in English, "Say it again."

Brazil was the place where Claude Lévi-Strauss carried out the very little fieldwork that was worked up into a theoretical contribution to structural anthropology, an anchor point in the 'structuralist' return to Freud that Lacan engaged in. Alongside the structuralist theories of language as a sign system in Ferdinand de Saussure's account of the distinction between signified and signifier as components of the sign, Lacan utilised Lévi-Strauss's analysis of underlying structures. These structures were organised around binary oppositions, between nature and culture, between the raw and the cooked, and between women and men, with women viewed as objects of exchange to guarantee the structured operation and separation of different kinship groups. Not only was the time Lévi-Strauss spent with indigenous peoples limited, he worked only with tribes in the Mato Grosso and part of Amazonia.

Things were very different in other parts of Brazil, the Rio-based anthropologist, Eduardo Viveiros de Castro, pointed out. If we were to take seriously what he called the 'Amerindian perspectivism' of the indigenous peoples of Brazil, Viveiros de Castro argued, then this would revolutionise our view of reality and subjectivity, with profound implications for psychoanalysis and politics. Instead of a strict separation between culture and nature, between human and non-human, Amerindian shamanic perspectivism includes, in different relational contexts, every object as 'human'. The conquistadors could not understand why they were able to make alliances at one moment with peoples they treated as less than human and then find those alliances broken when the indigenous peoples reinterpreted what really counted as culture and what as nature. The conquistadors, and succeeding generations of anthropologists from the West, including Lévi-Strauss, subjected the indigenous peoples to a narcissistic gaze in which they were viewed as being, in some way, albeit deficient, as like them. We assume that nature is universal and culture is particular, but Amerindian perspectivists reverse that; for them, culture is universal and nature is particular.

Viveiros de Castro turned to the so-called 'anti-Oedipal' cosmology of Gilles Deleuze and Félix Guattari, who, in their 1972 classic *Anti-Oedipus*, accused psychoanalysis of assimilating different kinds of experience to nuclear familial structures, effectively 'familialising' psychoanalysis. For Viveiros de Castro, a Deleuzian cosmology is anti-psychoanalytic; he is not interested in engaging with Lacanians, including critical Lacanians like Chris Dunker. We have, instead, to break from the Western colonialist structuralist preconceptions that subject peoples to one anthropological vision of what reality is and how each subject should be adapted to it.

Viveiros de Castro may be right, but whether his hostility to psychoanalysis as a reactionary relic of colonialism is fair or not is another matter. Among the diverse quasi-Lacanian groups in Brazil are followers of Deleuze and Guattari, and these acolytes were the most visible psychoanalytic contributors in sessions at the World Social Forum in 2002. It was extraordinary to see, amidst the indigenous and women's meetings and LGBT marches, sessions that were discussing the role of psychiatry, psychology and psychoanalysis in the alter-globalisation movement. The followers of Deleuze and Guattari argued for the construction of different 'assemblages' to bring about political change that was linked to transformations in subjectivity. They made no presuppositions about the nature of reality, for that reality was constructed through forms of culture, nor about forms of enlightenment as needing to be modelled on what had occurred in Western culture two hundred or so years before.

These psychoanalysts were working in the spirit of the World Social Forum, in line with the slogan of the Forum, that 'another world is possible'. You could not apply our models of subjectivity here. The 2002 visit was the first in a long series of exchanges and projects, which included translating Chris Dunker's work into English – articles and one of the first book-length historical surveys of the development of psychoanalysis from a radical Brazilian vantage point – and much later the translation of my book on Lacan into Portuguese by a group of students directed by him at Universidade de São Paulo, with critical input alongside organisation of meetings there by Ilana Mountian. The Brazilians taught us that psychoanalysis in different clinical and cultural contexts is not what we had been told it is. It never is, it is never what you think it is. Psychoanalysis in Brazil was something else.

14

TRAUMA

Truth and reconciliation

This chapter focuses on one attempt to draw together different attempts to 'apply' psychoanalysis, and to gather bodies from different traditions together in order to debate what this might look like. A living, breathing, flesh-and-blood laboratory was formed to explore whether psychoanalysis as a treatment of individuals can be 'applied' to collectives, institutions and societies, and we can see here conceptions of trauma, even the 'chosen trauma' of particular social groups. This putative application of clinical theory to social issues raises a deeper clinical and political question, whether psychoanalysis is a practice of reconciliation or one of bearing unending conflict.

Bodies

Sometimes, when I could not get to London, my supervision was on the phone. I knew of other people who had analysis by phone or by Skype, and there were rows inside the IPA in 2002 over telephone psychoanalysis, prompted by the practice of some of their members in South Korea. This, it was argued by the purists who insisted on face-to-face meetings between analyst and analysand, broke dramatically from Freud's own practice, though they conveniently overlooked the fact that some of Freud's analysands continued their analysis while out walking with him. I was told by a friend in Caracas that the traffic and travel conditions were so difficult across the Venezuelan capital that they sometimes saw their analysands in McDonalds.

The key, according to the mainstream IPA argument against the Koreans, was that physical proximity was crucial to the analytic process. The issue here is not so much 'face-to-face' analysis, because the technical device of the couch deliberately cuts that quintessentially imaginary channel of communication. Freud once said that he put his patients on the couch to talk into the air because he was fed up with them staring at him for ten hours a day, so this was another accidental discovery in the standard technique of psychoanalysis, like the fifty-minute hour as a function of particular personal lifestyle choices. The issue, something that has also been worried away at in the Lacanian tradition, where Jacques-Alain Miller has made a parallel argument to that made by the IPA, is not face-to-face but body-to-body.

It made a difference that I could hear Don's stomach gurgling after breakfast or Amelia slurping a cup of coffee in the evening, and I searched out every rustle and sigh behind me as evidence of agreement or impatience, things that would patch imaginary elements back into my speech echoing back to me from the Symbolic, from the particular version of the big Other I conjured into place when I spoke. Different psychoanalysts have intervened in this strange situation to different degrees over the years. When the psychologist Erik Erikson was in analysis with Anna Freud, he could hear the clicking of knitting needles behind him during the session, and when he announced the birth of his child she handed him a pair of little booties she had just finished in time. Amidst all the complaints about Lacan's infractions of psychoanalysis, ranging from varying the lengths of sessions to cutting his nails in another room during them to sleeping with his patients, the strange variations in practice in the IPA are usually overlooked. Erich Fromm married his analyst who was ten years older than him, and Wilhelm Reich was a repeat offender with his patients. Apart from the telephone crimes of the Koreans, and the many cases of analysts marrying their analysands, we read in the old analytic case studies of analysands being led into consulting rooms by the butler, not so bad, or sessions being brought to an end by a wife knocking on the door to tell the analyst that his dinner was ready, a bit weird.

The presence of the other's body gives an intimacy to the analytic encounter that makes the process of testimony on the part of the analysand so charged and the activity of bearing witness on the part of the analyst so draining. Psychoanalysis spread around the world rapidly between the world wars and contact between analysts was often by way of letters – with some of the most interesting ruminations about clinical and theoretical developments in Freud's work appearing in his correspondence with colleagues working in quite different conditions compared to those in Vienna. But the Wednesday seminars in Vienna, in which contributions to the discussion were decided by lot, by participants picking a piece of paper out of an urn to see who would speak next, and then congresses and then international congresses were absolutely essential to the moment-by-moment flow that body-to-body contact makes possible. Clinical case presentations often rely on direct bodily contact in order to bring about the illusion that the analysand is present again in the room and in the minds of the analysts.

With the fragmentation of psychoanalysis, its separation into different, distinct traditions with its own societies, seminars and congresses, bodily proximity also facilitates identification and corresponding hostility to the outsiders, against those who become enemies. The splits inside the societies, which produce factions and schools divided against each other, often function in much the same way as 'trauma' is described in psychoanalysis, with the temporal delay and retroactive self-recrimination that Lacan describes serving to intensify the schisms. An internal dispute, whether it is the latent hostility evinced by Lacan toward his own analyst, the ego-psychologist Rudolf Loewenstein, and then to the local apparatus of the IPA, or whether it is the suspicion on the part of Richard Klein that CFAR was straying from the path laid out by Jacques-Alain Miller as head of the WAP, often operates covertly initially.

The dispute operates as a breach in the collective self-image of the organisation, a breach in its ostensibly harmonious functioning, and exists for a while as a foreign body inside the organisation. Then something of the Real erupts, a Real as contradiction between different symbolic explications of what the difference is that is experienced as a Real outside the frame of discussion. It is often unclear to the host organisation exactly what this difference amounts to, where it will lead. And when the dispute erupts, it breaks the apparent understanding, the illusion of understanding, that had prevailed up to that moment, usually leading each party to the dispute, the host organisation and the now explicitly foreign body, to view each other as incomprehensibly other. The host body was toxic, it must be escaped. The foreign body is now revealed for what it always was, toxic, and it must be expelled. It is as if every psychoanalytic organisation is born from a traumatic moment that it worries over and re-characterises, reinterprets as an unwarranted expulsion, or, in the case of Lacan, an 'excommunication'. The moment is reinterpreted, functioning as an anchor point in the narrative of the group, as a kind of 'chosen trauma'. This phrase, 'chosen trauma', was coined by the IPA psychoanalyst Vamık Volkan to capture the way in which a people fabricates a history of the construction of national identity in a particular traumatic event or a series of events that are grouped together under a name, a signifier, that holds them together and makes them intelligible.

Recall Jean Laplanche's argument I described in Chapter 8, that in psychoanalysis it takes two traumas to make a trauma: an original undecipherable disturbance, fright or shock is buried in the unconscious, in this case in the narratives of historical folk memory, and is reactivated by a later event. The earlier event then becomes properly 'traumatic', something that was always there in the body that called to be voiced, and now it will be repeatedly voiced as a foundational element of the identity of the victim. It will be repeatedly voiced in the hysterical complaint of the analysand if it is not worried away at as an obsessional symptom, and will be repeatedly voiced in the collective entity that appeals to that event as evidence that it has the right to be a nation and to avenge its humiliating, wrongful, victim status. In this way the 'chosen trauma' plays a crucial part in the 'invention of tradition' that preoccupies the conscious activity of nations and individuals, accounting for how they have become who they are.

One of Volkan's most striking case examples is that of the 'chosen trauma' of the Serbs after Slobodan Milošević had an epiphanic moment in 1989 that transformed him from Stalinist bureaucrat into nationalist leader at the Gazimestan monument, site of the historical defeat of the Serbian nation in Kosovo in 1389. 1389 became the chosen trauma of the Serbs, redefining who they were, the identity of Serbia and all of the individual bodies that comprise the Serbian nation from that moment on, and from 1989 back. There was much discussion of Volkan's paper on Serbia inside group analysis, in which there were a number of IPA psychoanalysts active there, partly because the Institute of Group Analysis was beginning to expand its operations into ex-Yugoslavia after the fall of the Berlin Wall, and partly because the 'chosen trauma' motif was a way of bridging the gap between personal identity and collective identity, both now viewed as potent affectively-charged social constructions.

We, that is Erica and I, were discovering psychoanalysis around the world through our academic travels, sometimes through direct links with psychoanalysts who saw something psychoanalytic in the critical and qualitative psychology we were writing about, as was the case for Chris Dunker in Brazil, and sometimes through joint work around 'discourse analysis', through which we found colleagues interested in that methodology precisely because they were already also working psychoanalytically.

That was the case in South Africa, where we learned of the repeated attempts by the IPA to embed itself there as a training organisation, spending many thousands of pounds raised from local wealthy supporters to fund travel to London for personal analysis and training. In such instances, the IPA was willing to relax the five-times-a-week rule and South African analysands in training would fly backwards and forwards cramming their sessions into weekend blocks, rather like an individually-tailored tour version of the group analysis block trainings. The problem was that successful trainees who then became IPA analysts, people like the Kleinian Fakhry Davids, who was from the Cape Town Malay community, didn't go back. They stayed in London. There were also some Jungians in South Africa, buoyed up during the apartheid years by the racist, romantic ramblings of the pop-anthropologist Laurens van der Post.

There were also Marxist psychologists, such as Grahame Hayes in Durban, and 'critical psychologists', such as Derek Hook in Johannesburg, who were keen to follow through a discursive historical understanding of the construction of subjectivity by way of Lacan. I examined Derek Hook's PhD, and when Derek got a teaching post at the London School of Economics, LSE, there was an opportunity to take forward psychoanalytic work connected with politics, drawing on the resources of the LSE to bring together psychoanalytic researchers from around the world and even to make psychoanalysts from different clinical traditions speak to each other. I had also examined a number of PhDs at the LSE, which was an opportunity to get to know the students' supervisor Patrick Humphreys who, though trained as a social psychologist specialising in communication and media, had a long-standing personal and professional link with psychoanalysis.

Patrick Humphreys and Derek Hook at the LSE and Erica and I from Manchester began planning a conference as soon as I finished my training with CFAR. Erica had completed her group analytic training, and we knew that one of the advantages of bringing group analysis into the event was that it would also automatically link us not only with a generation of socialist and feminist activists who had journeyed into psychoanalytic practice but also with non-Lacanian psychoanalysts, both from the

IPA and also even from the Jungian tradition, some of whom were now beginning to characterise themselves as psychoanalysts rather than 'analytical psychologists'. We wanted to ground discussion of psychoanalysis in different political contexts, and we wanted to sidestep the linguistic or discursive debates that too quickly signalled to too many psychoanalysts that they were being drawn onto Lacanian territory. That is how we settled on the title for the conference, which took place in April 2005, 'Flesh and Blood'.

Flesh

How would we get all these bodies, some housing egos the size of planets, into the same room? And how would we enable dialogue across political divisions in which the different standpoints and forms of analysis were already in some cases diametrically opposed, even before we got to the disputes between different psychoanalytic traditions? We drew on the expertise of group analysts to think through the structure of sessions and to organise the discussions that took place on the evening prior and on the two days of the Flesh and Blood conference. That worked, up to a point, but you have to bear in mind here that group analysis, for all of the weight placed by supporters and detractors, mainly detractors, on its focus on 'ego training in action', is an approach very much in line with psychoanalysis as such.

Group analysis, as you have already seen, is a form of psychoanalysis, working on the assumption that we human beings are divided subjects, divided between consciousness and the unconscious, and radically divided at an unconscious level. This means that there is no reasonable hope for healing divisions but rather of arriving at a better understanding of how those divisions work. Group analysts working in consultancy roles, for example, do not, or should not, ever promise to make the organisation run more smoothly. Conflict is at the heart of the human subject, and so individually-focused psychoanalysis and group analysis each track that conflict and the way it manifests itself, the way it organises itself around symptoms, conflicts that are symptomatic of deeper interminable conflicts. The most we could hope for in Flesh and Blood would be for a tolerable degree of common unhappiness at the state of the world, at our impossible irresolvable relationship with political processes.

Opening the first evening was the feminist literary theorist Jacqueline Rose speaking about Israel and Palestine in a lecture called 'The Last Resistance', with responses by Farhad Dalal, who was now trained as a group analyst, Stephen Frosh from Birkbeck College and the Tavistock Clinic, and Renata Salecl from the Slovene School of Psychoanalysis. Jacqueline Rose's book *The Question of Zion* had just been published as one of a series of public interventions she had made supporting the Palestinians, and Stephen Frosh had also been actively involved in this question, questioning Zionism as the only legitimate expression of Jewish identity, and opening a space for Jews to organise independently of Israel, even against the Israeli state. What 'resistance' meant in this context, then, was loaded with ambiguity. The separate poster for Jacqueline Rose's lecture, with an image that she suggested for the lecture, was of the Separation Wall.

Some of those participating in discussion at the lecture, including Stephen Frosh, had been involved in 'reconciliation' initiatives in Israel and Palestine, where there had also been several attempts at combined group psychotherapy events run by group analysts. The question of conflict and reconciliation was a potent theme running through the following two full days of the conference, with detailed discussion of the peace process in the north of Ireland revolving around the 1998 Good Friday Agreement. Isabel Piper Shafir travelled from Chile to talk about a similar process following the fall of the Pinochet dictatorship, and Grahame Hayes described the work of the benchmark Truth and Reconciliation Commission, the TRC, after the end of apartheid in South Africa.

These discussions about the legacy of profound political trauma also brought us up against some of the limits of truth and reconciliation when the political conditions that had led to the conflict had not yet really been resolved. The South African TRC, for example, had, as Grahame pointed out, raised expectations that the process would not only reveal the truth about the atrocities that been committed by the regime as well as by the opposition, but would also in some way be 'therapeutic'. The TRC did not aim directly to be therapeutic, but this was the implicit promise that drew many people in to tell their stories and find others to bear witness. The TRC hearings corralled participants into speaking only about events that fitted with the remit of the commission, and back-door deals to encourage perpetrators to come forward and confess meant there were limits placed not only on the kind of compensation that victims were demanding but also on the time and value that was given to their testimony. Grahame argued that many participants had come away traumatised, silenced by the TRC because their stories did not correspond to what were expected and demanded. While it had been a bold political project it had failed at many levels, crucially at a personal level, at the level of subjectivity as it intersects with politics, there where the personal becomes political.

As well as Elisabeth Rohr from Germany and Erica from the organising team, there were a number of prominent group analysts present at all the sessions, including Sheila Ernst, Sue Einhorn, Dick Blackwell, Martin Weegmann and Isobel Conlon. This presence helped keep discussions on track, on a track that would include as many participants as possible while reflecting on the contributions. What also helped more than we had expected was the presence of scribes, led by Garrick Jones, who rapidly converted the spoken introductions to each session into graphic image representations on large whiteboards at the front of the room. We could then track what was being said and so we had a visual reminder of it throughout the discussion.

Blood

Flesh and Blood held itself together over the two-and-a-bit days it was scheduled for, just long enough for us to survive working together as a team. Some of the hidden agendas for the conference unravelled, and it took a while after the event to make sense of how we had failed as well as how we had succeeded. Erica and I were lured in, for example, by the promise of financial resources for the kind of event we never could have put on in Manchester, particularly at an ex-Poly, an ex-Poly that London-centric psychoanalytic folk wouldn't travel to, let alone international visitors. That worked out. It happened. But we were also lured in by other hints by Patrick Humphreys that the LSE was, as he put it, like a 'club', with people joining it not so much on the basis of job applications and interviews but on the basis of an experience of 'working together'.

We were sceptical because we had friends who had applied for posts and been interviewed at the LSE, but we played along, even, I suppose, took the bait as much as pretended to take the bait. We even at moments in the planning process and, in our morning journeys across the Thames from the LSE hall of residence where we stayed during the conference itself, wondered what it would be like to relocate from Manchester to London. Perhaps we could build a psychoanalytic base at the LSE, but we knew that if we did we would then be condemned to spending the rest of our lives with these difficult people, with the enmeshed inbred and warring psychoanalytic communities in the congested, overstuffed capital. We did, at any rate, get through the event well enough to be able to organise another international conference at the LSE a year later with existentialist Lacanian Simona Revelli and the new College of Psychoanalysts in the UK, which had been spear-headed by Jacques China and Haya Oakley, to bring together practitioners who declared themselves to be psychoanalysts without the imprimatur of the IPA. That later conference was 'Psychoanalysis and State Regulation', devoted to the threat by the British government to define who could call themselves a psychoanalyst and what they could do in their consulting rooms.

Behind the scenes, Flesh and Blood lurched from crisis to crisis making us feel that we never again wanted to repeat it, and plans for a book series based on the sessions never came to fruition. The first evening lecture was in crisis even before it happened: one speaker phoned that morning to ask how they were to get from north London to the LSE, and the administrator told them about the different bus and underground train options. But no, they said, "I don't travel by public transport." A taxi was arranged, and they did their talk very well.

Susie Orbach, one of the founders of the Women's Therapy Centre in London, turned up that evening before Jacqueline Rose's lecture to say that she had not written a paper for her session on the last day and that it might be better just to have a discussion. I spent the time while people were arriving for the lecture pleading with Susie to rethink, and perhaps at least say a few things before we went into discussion. I was sure we could arrive at some compromise if I could contain my anger, for we had gone through some such compromise arrangements a couple of years before when I invited her to write an article about her work with the Women's Therapy Centre for a special issue of the *European Journal of Psychotherapy, Counselling and Health* on 'Therapy from the Left: The Personal from the Political'. She was too busy to write an article, she said then, but would agree to be interviewed if I would travel down to London. I hadn't met her so I jumped at the offer and went down in November 2002. I had to work on the transcription of the interview, reordering and tidying up the scattered conversation we held at her apartment in Belsize Park, and then she did do a lot of work on it in time for it to appear in print a year later.

There was a discussion at Flesh and Blood of radical Slovene art practice by the curator and theorist Marina Gržinić and Alexei Monroe. Marina had been wary about attending the event because, she said, she had had a bad experience at another conference recently where she had been put in accommodation miles and miles away from the venue. I had met her at an event in Manchester the previous year where she had told me "Slavoj Žižek is my father," but when I looked surprised she qualified this saying, "I mean, of course, that I love him as my symbolical father." We found Marina a hotel near the LSE and she spoke at the event about the bizarre reappropriation of art from the era of the Russian Revolution by socialist and feminist activists in Slovenia, particularly work by the Suprematist Kazimir Malevich. I will tell you more about this, and what Žižek has got to do with it in the next chapter. We invited, as discussant for that session, the Jungian analyst Andrew Samuels who turned up with a large, rectangular, unwieldy package wrapped in brown paper. He unveiled it to reveal an original painting by Malevich. Andrew said his family in Liverpool had almost gone bankrupt and had to sell most of their paintings brought over from Eastern Europe, but had hung onto this one. "This is the original," he said brightly, to which Marina growled "we prefer the copies."

The journal special issue with the Susie Orbach interview also contained a review of a recent book by Andrew Samuels, something that I hoped would smooth over a rocky relationship that began with a critical review I had written for the journal *Feminism & Psychology* of his 1993 book *The Political Psyche*. I liked that book and said so, but Andrew thought I didn't like it enough, and took badly against the review, writing a letter to the journal editors saying so – also lobbing in the complaint that I had specified the theoretical orientation of my analyst, in another article elsewhere, as Anna Freudian. The journal editors must have been bemused. He had already angrily brandished a flyer for our Psychoanalytic Studies programme at a conference in London – I heard this from Erica who was distributing the leaflet – complaining that we were once again excluding Jung from psychoanalysis. He included this point in the letter of complaint, saying that the combination of Lacanian and IPA traditions in our course programme recalled the psychic defence that Anna Freud called 'identification with the aggressor'. When I first met Andrew, at a conference, he told me that he had been reading about Michel Foucault to try to work out where I was coming from that would make me so hostile to his book; it was an encounter he opened with the disarming, but not very reassuring, comment "I don't hate you." We got Andrew up to Manchester that year for a day conference on masculinity and psychoanalysis in which the other speaker was Carol Gilligan, a psychologist who hears a different ethics enunciated in the voices of young women. They each, Andrew and Carol, spoke as if from a pulpit, and different sections of the room murmured their appreciation as if in a gospel choir during their presentations. They each in their different ways linked ethics with politics.

Ethics is often a weasel-word in discussions among psy-practitioners, and when someone bangs on about how important it is to be 'ethical', as if it were about following the right rules carefully enough, then it is time to start counting your spoons; something is about to spill out beyond those rules, temptations to transgress them. In contrast with those who conflate ethics with morality, with a shared moral code that then weighs down on people and punishes them for infractions of it, Lacanians treat ethics as a reflexive engagement with what it is to speak, honouring difference, not expecting people to be the same as each other, not even expecting people to be the self-same. I was struck by the way that Chris Dunker addressed this question when we were with him in São Paulo, visiting his new house, discussing which room would be for his son Mathias and which for his daughter Nathalia. I commented that the room pegged for Nathalia was the larger, implying perhaps that this was an unequal arrangement. Chris looked puzzled and then burst out laughing, and said mockingly "Oh I get it, it would be *unfair*!". So, no to some kind of utilitarian ethics in which we balance out costs and benefits, ego work, or to common-sensical ideas of what is good and true, or to obedience to a moral command that would land us in the realm of the superego.

I must admit I was rather frustrated with the group therapy ethos that saturated some of the parallel group discussion sessions at Flesh and Blood, facilitated by practitioners with very diverse trainings – Karen Ciclitira, Simon Clarke and Jan Haaken – as well as in the main sessions where the analysts had an impossible task. The Lacanians, including Carol Owens, Rik Loose and Alan Rowan, had to fall in line with this therapeutic ethos, and so discussions oscillated between a desperate search for soothing agreement and some pretty sharp exchanges and political attacks. I wished for more robust political discussion – until things got very hot in an open conflict between Grahame Hayes and Sara Ahmed. "This is white theory," Sara snapped after Grahame's discussion of the context of the TRC in South Africa. This because Grahame, a Marxist, had pointed to the continuing inequality in South Africa under the new regime headed by the ANC (the African National Congress), and had argued that the new regime was perpetuating a version of apartheid in which the mass of the black population were still effectively disenfranchised, and that it was corrupt.

Erica and I knew well that Grahame Hayes, a white South African, had been politically active alongside the ANC under apartheid, and had worked therapeutically with victims of the security forces, and so we were completely unprepared, as was Derek Hook and as was Corinne Squire who had spent some time working in South Africa on different projects, for such a negative response to what Grahame was saying. I wondered if the dispute would spin into a conflict between male Marxists, insensitively criticising the government of a liberation movement, and feminists, attentive to dimensions of racism and, worse, cued into the 'hurt' that was being signalled by Sara Ahmed. Perhaps the very therapeutically-oriented types would be tempted to take things in that direction. On the other hand, there were socialist-feminists there, including Liz Bondi, Joanna Ryan and Lynne Segal, who were unlikely to let that happen.

The therapeutic frame to some of the discussions, including, of course, the therapeutic frame that promised that there could actually be shared, acknowledged 'truth' and a reconciliation of the conflicts that appeared between us – what Lacanians would view as in the line of the Imaginary – threatened to overwhelm not only the explicitly symbolic dimension that Sara Ahmed was clearly concerned with but also threatened to blot out the third dimension of the Real. The Real in this case had two aspects: first, the difficult, if not impossible, to symbolise material political-economic coordinates of the situation in South Africa, and, second, the irreconcilable conflict that expresses the position or standpoint of different political-economic groups.

The anthropologist Claude Lévi-Strauss had drawn attention to irreconcilable representations of the same community given by a dominant and subordinate group of Winnebago tribespeople in what is now the United States. The dominant group drew a circle with a line down the middle with them on one side, while the subordinate group draw a circle within a circle with them on the outside. The point Slavoj Žižek makes about this is that here there is no agreement over what the actual state of things is as a basis for discussion about how to resolve the contradiction: the very grounds of disagreement are contested. Here is the Real. Here too, we were at a deadlock. It was not resolved.

This description of what happened on those days at the LSE makes it sound like a huge conference, but there were less than a hundred people there in total, which added to the pressure. You will recognise the names of the usual suspects, those I have already mentioned in previous chapters, colleagues and friends in the rather tight-knit psychoanalytic community. There was greater opportunity for people who wanted to avoid each other to cross paths and clash. They did. That was Flesh and Blood, life on the edge: discussion about conflict interspersed with battles at lunchtimes to save the gluten-free dishes for those who needed them and the scooping out of the insides of sandwiches for those who were following the Atkins diet. This was the Real traumatic underside of academic life. In many contexts, you apply psychoanalysis at your peril. Well, I have mentioned Žižek already, so let us meet him now.

15

THEORY

Žižek, culture and the clinic

One of the most wide-ranging recent attempts to 'apply' psychoanalysis is to be found in the voluminous, contradictory output of the Slovene theorist, Slavoj Žižek. This is psychoanalytic social theory with a political bite, claiming to link Lacan with Hegel and Marx, something that many liberal psychoanalysts, and not a few radicals, worry is more a hindrance than a help to their work. I will describe what the hooks were in Žižek's writing for me, and my attempt to make sense of a melange of cultural and philosophical reference points, an attempt that included tackling Žižek himself about it.

Idealism

"If you put a gun to my head," Žižek said in Ljubljana in September 2003, "I would choose German idealism; this is what I am really interested in." A very satisfying answer, exactly in line with the final draft manuscript of my book *Slavoj Žižek: A Critical Introduction* that he held in his hands. I had argued that, for Žižek, Lacan was but a theoretical apparatus to read Hegel, and that Marxist discourse was little more than that, discourse, a discursive resource to flesh out by way of pop-cultural examples, illustrations of the way German idealist philosophy could be reread. This was the project, it seemed, and the confusing zigzag through different theoretical debates in Žižek's writing now made more sense. This was almost the end of the intense academic research I had been carrying out while completing my CFAR training, and so we have to backtrack a little now to those last few months of 2003 when I tracked Žižek down and eventually persuaded him to write a nice little blurb endorsing my book for Pluto Press.

I got hold of his email address from a friend in July, informed him I was writing the book, that the manuscript was nearly finished, and that I wanted to discuss it with him. No reply. I emailed him again with no success, and then with the help of Detective Google guessed that he would be in Ljubljana in the middle of September. I emailed him again telling him that I would be arriving on Wednesday 10th and leaving on Sunday 14th, asking him for his address to send him a final draft copy of the book. He immediately replied saying that he would meet me at the Grand Hotel Union on Thursday morning and that he would give me three mornings. That's the hotel I booked into for Wednesday night and where I met him the following morning, and on his advice moved to a much cheaper hotel for the next three nights, a single bare cell of a room to which I retreated each day to take Paracetamol for headaches brought on by time with a guy who speaks non-stop in one-to-one conversation as if he were addressing an audience of a thousand. I am not sure if he agreed to meet me because I signed my emails 'Professor', that's what he called me when we first met, or because I said I was a Marxist, or because I said I was completing the CFAR training as a Lacanian psychoanalyst.

He was clutching a copy of the book's manuscript when I met him in the hotel lobby. He commented that this was a ridiculously stupidly-priced hotel for bureaucrats and politicians, and told me that we should go to a traditional, "completely fascist", typical Slovene restaurant where they would serve food full of cream and fat that would cause a heart attack. That's where we went. I had soup and he had salad. Then we went to his apartment block, then up in the elevator while he complained about the old, squat barracks complex of Metelkova, which I said I had visited the previous night. "My enemies", he said. "They," he said, the anarchists and punks that had set up café bars and meeting spaces, "they say they are 'civil society', well, no, *this*," he gestured around him at his apartment block, "*this* is civil society." We were already thus immersed in a Hegelian conceptual universe in which 'civil society' is the necessary mediating realm between the family and the state, an invaluable realm for the production of reflexive, competent citizens that needs to be defended against petty, personal interests and against the bureaucracy. Metelkova, for Žižek, was both petty private enterprise and worse, he claimed, they took money from the state. He showed me his neatly-organised bookshelves, and then the doorbell rang; it was the postman with plane tickets for his forthcoming trip to South Korea. He anxiously tore open the envelope saying that he wanted to check that he was travelling first-class, because, he said, he wanted to see what was on the upper deck of the plane.

We sat in his kitchen and I set up my tape recorder, and took some photos of him. He fussed around opening and closing the refrigerator while muttering that he might have something there, but, no, it was empty, and that it was always good to keep the fridge empty to stop you from eating too much. He sat down and said "OK, you're the boss," before gasping and pointing to the window behind me exclaiming "My god, there is a man on the roof, an assassin with a gun; he is going to shoot us." There was indeed someone on the roof. Žižek sat down again and, as the tape recorder was already running, we began.

Žižek is the most prominent member of the Slovene Lacanian School, a group of scholars that had for many years been working through Lacan's texts in relation to different philosophical traditions, but mainly with reference to the German idealist tradition that has Hegel at the core. I had seen his ex-wife Renata Salecl in

Metelkova the previous night. "People say that I stole some of her ideas," he said one day, "but that is impossible, because," he clapped his hands in delight and leaned back, "I never read what she wrote!" A friend in Metelkova told me that I should talk to Rastko Močnik, one of the founders of the School who had now broken with Žižek, but I couldn't get a reply on the phone while I was there, and Žižek said I should "meet the guys", by which he meant Mladen Dolar and Alenka Zupančič, but that never happened. Otherwise he was a solicitous host, giving of his time and attention, eager to help, addressing me as a comrade.

There is already plenty of Hegel in Lacan. The master-slave dialectic permeates Lacan's account of the mirror-stage and then the operations of the Imaginary. The Symbolic is configured for each individual as the big Other to whom they are beholden, from which they crave recognition. And the Real as impossible exists in tension with the Imaginary and Symbolic, knotted together with them, but never actually comprehensible as such, always blocked and distorted by what Lacan calls the 'wall of language'. The word, Lacan declares, referring to Hegel, is 'the murder of the thing'; as we speak we betray, our words ineluctably drive us away from what we speak about in linguistic rhetorical processes that repeat Freudian themes: metaphor as repression, murder of the thing, and metonymy, the perpetual chase from signifier to signifier, in a search for the lost object of love, desire that covers over the traces of the crime. The structures that Lacan outlines in the four discourses, of master, university, hysteric or analyst, are driven by the same Hegelian concerns with recognition and misrecognition. The agent confronts the other, concealing the truth and producing something that is also emblematic of loss, whether that is the agent as master signifier, as knowledge, as barred subject or as *objet petit a*, the semblance of the lost object that elicits compelled confused desire from others.

What Žižek does so well is to remind us of other Hegelian conceptual underpinnings for fundamental psychoanalytic processes, of the Hegelian basis of psychoanalytic ontology and epistemology, of what we are and how we can come to know it. When we follow this return to Hegel, it is not only Freud but Lacan too that begins to make more sense. Not complete sense, of course, that would be very un-psychoanalytic – for that would turn psychoanalysis into something transparent to thought, turn it into what you think instead of something of the unconscious.

Žižek's Hegel turns the Freudian unconscious inside out, not only through the externalising of internal subjective processes so that it is then also possible to agree with Lacan that the unconscious is the discourse of the Other, but also by shifting focus from the positive energetic qualities of the unconscious to what always rebels, negates. While 'negation' for Freud lies on the side of the ego, it is one of the defence mechanisms, for Lacan, that becomes the decisive primal defence mechanism for the production of perverse clinical structure. For Žižek there is fundamental 'negativity'. The unconscious at the heart of the human subject is what Hegel once called 'the night of the world', radical negativity.

The twists and turns of the subject who refuses to acknowledge such negativity then include the Hegelian figure of 'the beautiful soul'; the hysteric who sees chaos and danger in the outside world and complains about that, complains about how that chaos and danger intrudes upon their own private space, is a beautiful soul. Hystericization of the subject in the clinic, the eliciting of rebellious complaint as a condition for the analysis to proceed and for something of the unconscious to be made present, must then always be accompanied by interpretative strategies that, in different ways, return to the same question; 'And you, what is it for you, where are you in this?'

One manifestation of this beautiful soul, and one that gives a neat Hegelian-Lacanian reading of charitable efforts to help victims and to ensure that the others we help stay victims so that we can continue to help them, is in what Žižek, after Hegel, calls 'the gaze that sees evil'. The gaze that sees evil in the world is itself evil, and one of the key lessons of psychoanalysis is that we are an integral part of the world we describe. There is no neutral, objective position from which we can describe social relationships, we are always implicated, our subjectivity enmeshed with the terrible things we rebel against and blame on others. Lacan insists that no metalanguage can be spoken. This Žižekian Hegel that links us to psychoanalysis is therefore also a potent social theory, specifying us as social beings whose very forms of knowledge sustains us as such.

On the first morning we didn't only talk about Hegel. We talked about everything at once. At least Žižek did. At the end of the first meeting, he said, "OK, tomorrow morning here, what about eight o'clock," and, when I blenched at that time, said "Oh I see, everything for the revolution except getting up early in the morning." We agreed to meet on Friday at nine. I left and went and moved to my cheaper hotel, and took some headache tablets and had a rest.

Materialism

Ernesto Laclau, who, with Chantal Mouffe, introduced Žižek to the English-speaking world, warns readers in his preface to Žižek's 1989 classic text *The Sublime Object of Ideology* published by the leftist publishers, Verso, that this is no ordinary book, it does not even have the structure that one would expect of a book. Žižek, in this book, and through the following ones that he pumped out at a rate of about one a year, circles around a series of philosophical problems in German idealism that connect Lacan with Marx. In some ways this reference to Marx and Marxism is hardly surprising. Žižek was steeped in Marxist social theory through his early university career in Yugoslavia, even though he was viewed as too untrustworthy by the regime to be awarded a lectureship at the University of Ljubljana, and went on to do postgraduate research in Germany on the Frankfurt School, his first intellectual stop in psychoanalytic post-Marxist study before arriving at French structuralism. More than that, he worked for a subcommittee of the League of Communists of Slovenia, taking minutes of meetings and even at times contributing to speeches by apparatchiks that he could then deconstruct, submit to a critical reading. He was on the edge of the regime, but an insider to it, and played with this liminal role, taunting communist and anti-communist political activists when Yugoslavia crumbled toward the end of the 1980s, reminding them of his links to the apparatus and telling them he was never really signed up to it.

What is crucial here is neither the claim that he really was complicit as clerk and sometime speech-writer in the crimes of Stalinism in this northernmost part of Yugoslavia nor that he had an authentic history of dissident activity working against the regime. Rather, it is the process of dissimulation that riddles the position of both sides of the story that bothers him and that he worries away at; suspicion that those who parrot the official line never really believed it, that they conjured up an 'Other' for whom they performed their belief; and contempt for the 'dissidents' who were permitted to grumble about the bureaucracy as long as they never actually did anything about it, who let things carry on.

Remember that for Freud, the key to the interpretation of dreams is not the hidden secret meaning of the dream itself, as if we could dredge up the unconscious and make it completely visible, still less make the unconscious conscious and heal the division between these two realms of the speaking subject. The key is the 'dream-work'; not what is repressed, but how the repression is incessantly repeated. Repression as such is never something that is accomplished once and for all, then to be forgotten. Repression is ceaseless, exhausting, a continual process of pushing away what the subject does not want to think about. The first chapter of *The Sublime Object of Ideology* revolves around Lacan's cryptic comment that Marx invented the symptom, and Žižek's explication of this is by way of a 'fundamental homology', as he puts it, between dreams as interpreted by Freud and commodities as analysed by Marx. At this point Marxism in Žižek's writing is not just a discursive resource; Žižek is intervening in it and showing us something new.

As with the analysis of a dream, Marx is clear that the task is not to arrive at the 'hidden kernel', not to unveil exactly what a commodity is as such. Rather, the task of Marxist analysis is to show how human labour under conditions of exploitation and the extraction of surplus value from workers by their employers comes to take the form of a commodity. A commodity, Marx points out in the first volume of *Capital*, is such a mysterious thing precisely because it is there that the social character of labour is 'stamped upon' its product, as if it were an objective thing. This commonality between dreams and commodities has practical consequences for how both can be conceptualised and unravelled.

In psychoanalysis, for example, if the 'dream' was a finished product that simply needed to be deciphered, then the best person to do it would be the psychoanalyst who would know what the meanings really were. It is precisely because the dreamwork is the focus, the *process* of concealment, the real concern of psycho-analysis, that the analyst must catalyse the speech of the analysand so that they are the ones who 'interpret'. In the process of interpretation they make themselves present as 'subject of the enunciation' rather than subject of the statements that experts might make about what images and narratives their patients have turned up at the clinic with. Just as it is the process of concealment that is crucial in the production of dreams, the repression as such, so it is the process of speaking that is crucial to their dismantling.

For Marxists, there is a correlative process. The commodity is not there to be unwrapped so that we can discover what its hidden kernel is. That was the mistake of classical liberal economists that Marx argued against, and that is why *Capital* is a critique of classical political economy. Instead, the process by which work is transformed into the commodity is what is at issue, a transformation that can only be grasped and unravelled in the 'praxis', the combined theory and practice of workers themselves. One of the reasons Žižek is attentive to that distinction between top-down and authentic mutative interpretation and action by the subjects themselves, I suspect, is because he was brought up under a regime that called itself Marxist but which arrogated to itself the expertise to tell its citizens what this meant. The Frankfurt School, and then other versions of Hegelian-inflected readings of Marx, emphasised the self-activity of the working-class, a more authentic version of the so-called 'self-management' style of bureaucratic state control that was trumpeted by the apparatus in Belgrade and then closer to home in Ljubljana.

Hysterical symptoms are defined by way of a process of 'conversion' in which one kind of conflict, a conflict between a desire and the forces that prevent that desire from being spoken, is displaced, translated into another kind of conflict, usually a somatic complaint in which a part of the body that is charged with meaning is paralysed. The obstruction of function now takes place in the body, with the meaning of this bodily complaint effectively hidden, alienated from the subject. Obsessional neurotic versions of this displacement have the conflict reproducing itself in thoughts rather than in the body, in rumination and procrastination. Marx invented the symptom, Žižek claims, when he traced the way that relations of power are 'repressed' under capitalism so efficiently that all involved are able to convince themselves that everyone is free and equal. Commodities appear to operate as a relation between things instead of as a social relationship. Social protest can then take different 'symptomatic' forms in which they speak of exploitation, expressing the conflict present under capitalism, but cryptic. Just as hysteria speaks of repression, so such deflected class struggle speaks of oppression.

For Marx there is a materialist substrate of the ideological illusions that are so efficient in misleading people over the causes of their distress under capitalism, the mode of production that relies on the extraction of surplus value and the circulation of commodities. What Žižek is most concerned with, however, is analysis of those ideological illusions. Instead of locating 'false consciousness' as individual misunderstanding inside individuals, there is what the Marxist economist Alfred Sohn-Rethel, writing on the edge of the Frankfurt School about intellectual and manual labour, calls 'necessary false consciousness', part of the structure of ideology as such. Illusion, Žižek insists, is not on the side of knowledge but of reality itself, of what people are perpetually doing to reproduce capitalist relations. Reality itself, as Lacan points out, is infused with fantasy; we open our eyes after a night's sleep so we can carry on dreaming with our eyes open.

Friday lunchtime, after meeting at Žižek's apartment, he walked me around his old stamping ground; here the building where he had to check in to write the committee meeting minutes, and around the corner the cinema where he could spend time during the day watching films from the West, those that he writes about before he goes back to the office to check out at the end of a day's work. So, he was part of the regime, yes? He laughed, and repeated a joke he had often made publicly before, which is that the only position he would take up in government in Slovenia would be as Minister of the Interior or Head of the Secret Police.

Structuralism

Žižek is allergic to psychoanalysis in the clinic, he told me. He was six months in analysis with Jacques-Alain Miller, but he left abruptly, then posted the outstanding payments in cash, and that was that. In other interviews he has often claimed that he went to Miller with ready-made dreams so he had something to talk about, a typical obsessional strategy for avoiding speaking the truth.

Nevertheless, whether or not we describe it as transference, there is powerful lingering allegiance to Miller, and Žižek's characterisation of Lacanian psychoanalysis is filtered through Miller's own reading, which often focuses on the 'later Lacan' and the Real. Even in *The Sublime Object of Ideology*, the second chapter traces a shift in Lacan's work from the symptom as simultaneous expression and dissimulation of conflict to the 'sinthome', a knotting of the Symbolic, Imaginary and Real that Lacan described very late on, in his 1975–1976 Seminar XXIII. This knotting of the three registers of the human being as a speaking being is singular, specific to each subject. Here Žižek risks laying out Lacan's contribution as if it formed one discrete theoretical framework, a structuralist account of a psychoanalyst whose work, as Žižek points out in many other places, continually mutated in an innovative self-correcting process of the reading and rereading of Freud.

Here there is a tension between the legacy of a hard-line, determinist, structuralist reading of Freud and Lacan, which one finds in some of Miller's early work, and a more rebellious anarchic characterisation of desire and of rupture of symbolic coordinates in 'act' that Žižek looks to as a way out of an ideological system, even sometimes as a way out of ideology altogether. Miller's induction into psychoanalysis and the work of Lacan was through Louis Althusser, who, with his account of the 'interpellation' or hailing of subjects into ideology by way of the Ideological State Apparatuses, functioned much of the time through his membership of the French Communist Party as a Stalinist 'philosopher of order', as Jacques Rancière put it. One of Miller's first theoretical papers on psychoanalysis, written in 1964 as a member of a Lacanian 'cartel' working on the topic of 'discourse', was called 'Action of the Structure'. This, note, was the year that Lacan was finally 'excommunicated' by the IPA and set up his own psychoanalytic school. Here, in this paper, Miller argues that individual 'experience' is illusory, imaginary, that which is worried away at by psychology, something that you could say reappears in Žižek's work as 'the sublime object of ideology'.

Žižek's analyses of racism as a centrepiece of ideology are also indebted to Miller, particularly the motif of the 'theft of enjoyment', analysis of the way that an 'other' is positioned simultaneously as being too lazy and as working too hard, as the site of an enjoyment that must, the racist subject presumes, have been stolen from them. Here Žižek extends psychoanalytic analyses of antisemitism as an integral part of capitalist ideology, analyses that appear in different forms throughout his work and that have an uneasy relationship with his take on Hegel and what he calls the 'Christian legacy'. There is an oscillation in Žižek's writing, which is very clearly expressed in his political interventions, and even more so in statements that are clearly designed as exaggerated provocations, statements that speak something of the truth of his position, something more than he would like to admit.

On the one hand there is a pessimistic assessment of the development of capitalism as the only imaginable system of rule. He often refers, for example, to *objet petit a* as the lure and obstacle to full freedom under capitalism, a lure and obstacle that is inherent to the system and a necessary condition of its perpetual revolutionising of society and subjectivity. Leftists, he claims, are bewitched by the fantasy that this lure and obstacle can be removed, as if there could be pure freedom. As a flip side to this reluctant acceptance of capitalism, there is repeated reference to Stalinism, in jokey asides, as a positive phenomenon. We spoke those mornings in Ljubljana about the psychoanalytic author Adam Phillips, for example, and of his books with large text and large margins; terrible; "to the Gulag with him", Žižek chuckled. Well before his recent calls for a strong charismatic figure to lead us out of crisis, 'a Thatcher of the left', he was disappointed that I had negative things to say about Hugo Chávez in Venezuela, and referred with admiration to Jacques-Alain Miller as "a master", and as a "Stalin figure".

On the other hand there is a fantasy of revolt, hysterical rebellion through 'act' that would, he claims, change the symbolic coordinates of a society. If we were to indulge in a little reductionist psycho-pathographical analysis here, we could say that Žižek is a perfect hysteric, not the obsessional he claims to be, desperate for there to be a master so that he can depose it. I hesitate here, emphasising that it is 'as if' he is a hysteric, bearing in mind the number of psychoanalytic colleagues who said to me that Žižek is psychotic or a pervert. I am as unhappy with such quasi-psychiatric diagnoses as I am sceptical about the hidden existence of everlasting psychotic or perverse clinical structures.

My book about Žižek was published in 2004, and, at the launch events in Manchester and Dublin, I told an anecdote from the friend who had given me Žižek's email, an anecdote that then circulated on social media. You will see in a moment why I protect this friend's identity. In this anecdote, Ernesto Laclau phones Žižek during a political crisis in Slovenia before the fall of the old regime. Žižek tells Laclau that there is a terrible clampdown on dissent, and worse, that the regime is appointing political commissars in every workplace to ensure discipline and obedience. Laclau is shocked. But the good news, Žižek says, is that "in my workplace I am the commissar". I wanted to capture something of the hysterical position he adopts, and his playful references to the Stalinist apparatus.

Five years later, 2009, my book was translated into Slovene, and here there was a double problem. First, as my comrade Nik Jeffs in Ljubljana pointed out, Žižek's politics is nuanced very differently inside Slovenia from outside it. Inside Slovenia his politics are more on the side of order, Žižek himself standing for the Liberal Democrats in the presidential elections in 1990, for example, on a political programme that included neoliberal economic 'shock therapy' and the return of the death penalty. Outside Slovenia, as we know, he sometimes speaks as a Marxist, a revolutionary true to his previous allegiance to Maoist alternatives to Tito. Nik in Metelkova, back in 2003, had warned me that Žižek would be hostile to the unruly far-left opposition to the regime gathered in that area near his apartment block; "I am one of his enemies," Nik smiled. Now in 2009 I stayed in Nik's apartment to be ready to launch the book in Ljubljana, and Nik warned me: "you are a pawn in a bigger game."

The second problem was that Igor Vidmar, the publisher of the book, was one of Žižek's other enemies; ex-punk music agent Igor clearly relished the opportunity to attack Žižek. Igor, who had been imprisoned twice under the old regime, organised the book launch in the Ministry of Interior building in Ljubljana. He translated and circulated my initial launch piece with the anecdote joke about Žižek saying he was the commissar, and Žižek went up the wall. I was interviewed for newspapers and television while I was there, but already, before Žižek publicly responded to the launch piece, I was told that there were past students of his who were now working as journalists and those with links to the Slovene Lacanian School who kept away, refused to cover the story.

I was in a small world of political-theoretical rivals with old grudges, and I guess also that Žižek was genuinely worried, worried, as he said when he accused me of 'postmodern cynicism', that being linked to the old regime was dangerous, as I should know well. He knew well what barbs hurt most. We had disputes between 2004 and 2009, but this was the sharpest break. Žižek doesn't return my emails now, and I am clearly in the camp of his enemies. We are no longer in the realm of simple, abstract application of psychoanalysis but implicated in it, and that brings us to practical interventions in culture and politics in Slovenia.

16

IDENTIFICATION

Laibach and the state

We are moving beyond 'application' of psychoanalysis in this chapter, pushing at the limits of imposing a theoretical grid onto reality. Here I examine the way that psychoanalytic ideas have been put into practice outside the clinic, focusing on the cultural-political work of art collectives in Slovenia that employed notions of transference and 'over-identification' to challenge the regime, a challenge that then inspired some new theoretical movements inside psychoanalysis.

Identity

The Adria Airways brochure in the seat pockets of the plane from Manchester to Ljubljana had its back-cover page devoted to the group Laibach, a sign of their rehabilitation I guessed, very different from the old socialist days in Yugoslavia when they were banned simply for adopting that German occupation force name for the capital. Formed in 1980, the year of Tito's death, in Trbovlje in Slovenia's coal-mining region, Laibach were the most prominent of the wave of punk protests that kick-started the opposition to Stalinist rule. Notorious, Slovenia's equivalent to the Sex Pistols, but better, with television appearances set up to denounce them as fascists, they indeed dressed like fascists, always parading in uniform, never letting the mask slip throughout the 1980s, masters of deception. I was sure they actually were fascist.

My first night in Metelkova, site of one of their fan bases, was spent arguing with Nik Jeffs, an anarchist and sometime art curator, and Alexei Monroe, Laibach fan and theorist-advocate. I knew Laibach were fascist, with skinhead followers in East Germany, and with a penchant for German as their favoured album-track language. They had spent time in London in exile, and played in clubs where their audiences were divided between supporters of the neo-Nazi National Front and activists in Rock Against Racism and the Anti-Nazi League. There were fights. "Yes, yes, that's the point," Alexei said, "there is no agreement over what they are, but that does not mean they are fascist." You have to fight it out. Žižek said they took money from the state. I bought their latest album, *WAT*, which signifies 'We Are Time', before I left Ljubljana and played it when I got home. The track 'Tanz mit Laibach', dance with Laibach, was disturbing. I still wasn't sure Alexei was right about this.

By the time we got to the launch for my Žižek book in 2004, I had been won over, and I played 'Tanz mit Laibach' at a joint event in Manchester, where Alexei talked about NSK, Neue Slowenische Kunst, the art movement that Laibach were part of. One of the other components of NSK, the art collective IRWIN, had an exhibition that coincided with the book launch, and we had a bizarre dinner on the top floor of the gallery – with the guys from IRWIN dressed in their trademark sinister black suits and Marina Gržinić, who was working with the gallery on a 'new feminisms/new Europe' project. The dinner table was just round the corner from a mock-up of Suprematist artist Kazimir Malevich, low-lit in his coffin, mausoleum tribute-style. I asked the guys straight out about their politics. They answered that they had been brought up as working-class socialist youth. Erica asked them why the black suits and they said they wanted to look like Romanian businessmen.

The NSK cultural-political project was initially – in the 1980s as the regime was beginning to disintegrate – aimed at the assertion of identity in conditions where that was quite impossible, at a time when Slovenia was a subordinate partner in the Socialist Federal Republic of Yugoslavia. Neue Slowenische Kunst, German, of course, for New Slovenian Art, patched together the identity of the nation as every individual patches together their own personal identity, from the outside. Just as the ego for Freud is little more than an assemblage of images, identification with those we loved and hated, so this nation would, in NSK's mocking style, borrow from other cultures. Black Cross and Black Square Suprematist symbolism from Malevich was one instance – intense, explicit identification with a figure hailed by the new Soviet regime in 1917 as an artist of the revolution, when he did not support it, and a Russian icon when he was actually Ukrainian.

In 1987, NSK through its Novi kolektivisme group submitted the winning poster for Yugoslav Youth Day, which, not coincidentally, was also Tito's birthday. The poster was praised by the panel for showing the authentic character of Yugoslav socialist youth, until it was revealed that NSK had adapted their design from a Nazi poster from the 1930s. The issue of the radical weekly magazine *Mladina*, which carried an image of the poster was then banned. What these art interventions do is to make the process of identification explicit and rub the imagery that the apparatus of power uses to symbolise its domination in its own face, and in the process of adopting the imagery of power and 'détourning' it, much as the French Situationists would, tweaking the image, implicit subtexts are forced to the surface. The Yugoslav regime that claimed to stand as a monument to anti-fascist struggle was thus shown to rely on the self-same symbolic apparatus. So, to claim that Laibach is fascist is indeed to miss the point. This application of psychoanalysis makes visible the dreamwork of the political apparatus, showing how certain forms of power require certain forms of repression.

This intense and disturbing identification with power is termed 'over-identification', and there was some dispute between Žižek's followers and Laibach fans as to whether Žižek simply theoretically elaborated the already-existing art-political interventions of NSK, or whether NSK took up Žižek's ideas and turned them into practice. When Žižek describes over-identification in early English-language texts like *The Sublime Object of Ideology*, he very clearly identifies Laibach as the best example of the practice. However, there have been tensions between him and Laibach over the years, and in papers immediately after 2009: at this time he was annoyed at Igor Vidmar's publication of the translation of my book, and he refused to contribute to another edited book on the history of punk resistance that Igor was editing. Žižek then wrote about the German band Rammstein as being the best example of how to turn the stuff of ideology into nonsense, even though there is no political subtext in Rammstein's performances. Laibach say that they are Rammstein for grown-ups.

NSK art practice entails a particular kind of relationship to time that is very psychoanalytic. NSK takes up the 'retroactive' nature of time in psychoanalysis, the reconfiguring of traumatic past events in relationship to present-day trauma, to formulate its project as 'Retro-Avant-Garde'. It sidesteps the linear conceptions of many art movements in which there is, for example, a supposed transition from 'modern' to 'postmodern', in order to show how the past is always actually or potentially present. This is why Kazimir Malevich is such an exemplary figure, plucked out from a time of revolutionary transformation in Russia, his Black Cross and Black Square repetitively inserted into the different IRWIN artworks and used on the Laibach album covers and uniforms, uniforms that are Second World War US Air Force gear.

Over-identification took on a different dimension after Slovenia declared independence in 1991, and NSK State in Time was born as a direct, sarcastic response to this nationalist event. NSK State is sometimes described as a 'micro-nation', one of the many tactical political and cultural pretend-states that have sprung up, sometimes to defend refugees, sometimes simply as a joke launched on the internet from someone's bedroom. This state is not so small, however, claiming more citizens than the Vatican State, a significant comparison made from a country that, unlike Orthodox Christian Serbia to the south, is mainly Catholic. And it is a more ambitious and well-resourced project, producing convincing passports printed on paper smuggled out of Slovenia's own passport office. These passports, and citizenship, are available to anyone who applies regardless of geographical location; this is a 'State in Time' not in space, hence the Laibach track and album 'We Are Time'. So convincing were the passports that people used them to escape from Sarajevo in 1995 after NSK set up a consulate in the city.

The different components of NSK State in Time include the State Artists, that is IRWIN, the State politicians, that is Laibach, and the State Church, the Scipion Nasice Sisters Theatre, sometimes running under the names Red Pilot and sometimes as Cosmokinetic Theatre Noordung. There may be 14,000 citizens, but there is a very small 'members' group, and NSK are quite explicit that their regime is not democratic. How could it be? The forms of state in geographical territory that it over-identifies with are not themselves really democratic, and NSK is exaggerating, sending the truth back in reverse, in true form, about the nature of the different existing states that host it. State consulates, which pop up as art installations around the world, are bureaucratic machines.

My diplomatic passport was issued at a consulate in Thessaloniki in Greece, I already had a standard citizen's passport, and I remember well Lacanian political theorist Yannis Stavrakakis's exasperation at the ridiculous, drawn-out process of posing for passport photos and then waiting for IRWIN, still in their black Romanian-businessmen suits, slowly typing out the forms on old typewriters. It is amazing how quickly one can reproduce the Kafkaesque atmosphere of a real visa consulate in a small art space when people are desperate to get a passport, to get acknowledgement from this big Other, that they are recognised as citizens of this state. This assumed pretend-identity is itself absurd, of course, but what a lesson it is about identity as such, to be drawn into a machine that replicates what Althusser called the 'interpellation' of the subject by ideology in such a way as to deconstruct it.

Transgression

Laibach and NSK play with the pleasure of power, of over-identifying with power, and with the fantasy of transgressing power, a fantasy that is so potent in movements of resistance. Laibach know from attending Žižek's lectures when they were fine-art students, and from their time living in the basement of his house, that transgression is a necessary lure, correlative to prohibition. We desire to be free, and every attempt to clamp down on that freedom fuels the injunction to be free as a fantasy that, were it not for the busybodies and spoilsports, we tell ourselves and anyone else who will listen, we would have everything that we want and be completely happy. Psychoanalysis teaches us that the human condition is not suited to happiness, that the most we can hope for is the transformation of hysterical misery into common unhappiness, as Freud comments in one of his own gloomy but realistic recommendations for it as a treatment.

Lacan supplements this insight with the warning that fantasy functions as much as a shield against the deathly, self-destructive enjoyment, which he names '*jouissance*', as a yearning for satisfaction when we unconsciously stage our desire. We want everything, but it is a measure of our accession to the Symbolic that we are able to learn that we cannot have it, that there is a necessary limitation, a lack. This is a limitation that we first encounter in the manifestations of the Law of the Symbolic, which Lacan, in a typically patriarchal metaphor that threatens to prescribe what he describes, formalises as the metaphorical substitution of the Name of the Father for the Desire of the Mother.

What Laibach also know from their absorption of the 'French theory', which was such a powerful resource for the opposition movement in Slovenia in the 1980s – a cultural phenomenon that Žižek himself is one expression of – is that the dialectic between sadism and masochism that psychoanalysis explores in the clinic is neatly described in Michel Foucault's analyses of the institutional and cultural relationship between discipline and confession. Where there is power there is resistance, Foucault argues, and here he also has an eye to the intimate historical connection between domination and subjection, both of which are configured as enjoyable for those who participate in either side of the process or who oscillate between the two, oscillation that is the condition of the psychoanalytic subject, subject of the unconscious.

So tight were the connections between NSK and political movements in Slovenia that quite a few of the members of the new state apparatus after 1990 remained sympathetic to their old comrades. These personal-political connections were expressed in the promotion of Laibach in airline publicity and in exhibitions staged of IRWIN artworks in Ljubljana's galleries, and, in 2005, with the blessing of Slovenia's ambassador to Ireland, in the celebration of Slovenia's turn at the head of the European Union with a series of NSK events in Dublin. NSK issued passports at a consulate in Temple Bar, and the theatre group staged 'Supremat' at the Helix Theatre, which celebrated the contribution of Herman Potočnik-Noordung, an early twentieth-century Slovene army officer, to space travel.

At the Laibach concert it struck me, as I saw the shining, smiling faces of Alexei and NSK mates in the audience, that these really are fans. Alexei smuggled us into the after-show party where the disappointingly short Laibach guys lounged around in normal clothes and the seemingly muscular women, with blonde plaited-hair, who had been banging the drums Teutonic-style on stage, relaxed and talked about their PhDs on post-structuralism and pornography.

Laibach focus not on what has actually been repressed, but draw attention to the process of repression, not aiming to excavate and bring to the surface the real contents of the fantasy dreamscape of bourgeois ideology but showing us the dreamwork itself. This is real psychoanalysis. This is targeted at the operation of ideology as it simultaneously covers over and incites us to want all the more what is denied us; this is the heart of consumer culture, eliciting desire for lost objects and encouraging us to believe we can purchase them. This injunction to enjoy, for Lacan and then Žižek, is pure manifestation of the superego. This is what Laibach sarcastically play with, as they play with their audience, as they over-identify with the symbolic apparatus of power, and as they remind us how much we enjoy our submission and pretend-transgression of that apparatus even at the same moment as we declare ourselves to be repelled by it.

What about sex? Surely, if psychoanalysis is at work in NSK art-practice, then mobilisation and critique of the superegoic injunction to enjoy should have something to say about the way in which sex is targeted as the core of our being in consumer culture, the way that sexuality is commodified, turned into sex. Indeed it does, in the feminist NSK installations curated and theoretically elaborated by Marina Gržinić. At the 2001 Venice Biennale, Tanja Ostojić shaved her pubic hair into a square, that's Malevich's Black Square, and paraded around with an older, prominent male curator in a performance work called 'I'll Be Your Angel'. He was annoyed when he found out that he was merely a component in an artwork. At one of the events at the 'new feminisms/new Europe' series in Manchester in 2004, Ostojić came onto the stage dressed in a camouflage-pattern full burqa and shiny red high-heel shoes; she then described her art-project 'Looking for a Husband with an EU Passport'. In that project she sent out a naked photo of herself, inviting potential partners in Western Europe to hook up with her. She collated the replies, eventually engaging in a staged 'marriage' with a West German performance artist, which then traced through the process by which she could be recognised by the authorities to be a real wife, real in the eyes of the state.

What should be noticed here is that these performances of power and patriarchy do not, as analyses of the 'authoritarian personality' issuing from the tradition of the Frankfurt School do, reduce social practices to individual predispositions. Much as the work of the Slovenian Lacanian School and Neue Slowenische Kunst is indebted to the same two key theoretical resources that underpinned the Frankfurt School, that is Hegel and Marx, though they combine those two resources with psychoanalysis in quite a different way. On the one hand, there is a different evaluation of the historical process of personality formation under capitalism, and, on the other, there is thorough-going critique of what happened to the Frankfurt School when it got entangled in the adaptationist logic of émigré psychoanalysis in the United States.

The Frankfurt School analysis of the 'dialectic of Enlightenment', remember, traces a narrative in which Western civilisation reifies human collective, creative activity and desire, in which it sells those things back to the individual consumer as commodities. This grim linear developmental process is not, as we know Jürgen Habermas pointed out, very dialectical, for it is difficult to find grounds for hope in it. It eventually bears fruit in the United States in the pessimistic analysis of a 'culture of narcissism' advanced by Christopher Lasch, an analysis that was enthusiastically adopted by the *Free Associations* project in Britain. What Lasch then does, and this is where his description of the ills of capitalism twists into a prescription for patriarchy, is to nostalgically look back to a time before the family had been undermined by consumer culture, a hetero mythical time when individual men and women had the integrity to combine together to challenge capitalism.

One of Žižek's first English-language pieces, three years before the publication of *The Sublime Object of Ideology*, was a translation of a 1986 essay called 'Pathological Narcissus as a Socially Mandatory Form of Subjectivity', which appeared in the Croatian edition of Lasch's book, *Culture of Narcissism*. The essay draws attention to the first theoretical backdrop to his analysis, the Frankfurt School, including, at its edge, the energetic romantic theories of Wilhelm Reich as well as the reactionary dynamic of Lasch's argument. NSK's Retro-Avant-Garde approach, in contrast, refuses any such sentimental fantasy about returning to the past and retrieving what we have lost. It is more thoroughly psychoanalytic: we are divided subjects struggling to make sense of how we should construct ourselves as human beings.

When the Frankfurt School theorists, Adorno and Horkheimer, fled Nazism for the United States, they took with them a series of analyses of the way that authoritarian social practices fed fascism and antisemitism. Their analyses were of the profound cultural antecedents to the rise of Nazism – a peculiar contradictory combination of mysticism and technocracy – as well as analyses of the way that the Nazis displaced attention from the internal contradictions of capitalism onto the paranoiac image of the Jew as external enemy; this latter analysis is repeated by Žižek. Like many other émigré practising psychoanalysts, however, Adorno and Horkheimer adapted themselves to US culture, adapted themselves well enough to the very consumer culture they despised, but also adapted their research to empirical, positivist social science. This social scientific analysis focused on 'authoritarian personalities' with the aim of promoting a healthily-adapted 'democratic personality' for good citizens. In contrast, the last thing NSK can be accused of is promoting democratic good behaviour. Their interventions are designed to undermine conformity of any kind, whether that is authoritarian conformity of the right or good, comradely conformity of the left.

Having said that, NSK have themselves come under some ideological pressure to be well-behaved, and have flirted with democracy. The question is whether this is in line with psychoanalysis or a betrayal of it. Take the NSK 'Citizen's Congress' in Berlin in 2010. This assembly of 'citizens' was convoked by the IRWIN art-group, though members of Laibach also attended. I was invited to convene one of the parallel-session working groups, with strict instructions not to give my own analyses of the current state of NSK, rather to facilitate a small group of about fifteen people, citizens who had been specifically invited because of their long-standing links to NSK. Their assigned task was to suggest how NSK State in Time might be reformulated in a contemporary capitalist world, a world in which the old Stalinist regimes it had been designed to combat had all but disappeared. Participants had their travel and accommodation paid for from a European Union grant for the project, one paradox among many in the congress, and one that brought back to mind Žižek's complaint that these people took money from the state.

The focus-group ethos of the congress also jarred with the earlier pronouncements that NSK State is not democratic. There was some agonising over the uptake of NSK passports in Nigeria where they had been sold by unscrupulous middlemen to citizens who thought that they would be able to get to Europe with them. My group and the other three parallel groups dutifully shared ideas, respected each other's opinions, and prepared flip-chart lists of proposals for the future direction of the state, which were then shared in a plenary session. Laibach were not impressed, announcing in the final plenary session that they were, they said, "orphans of the state". Since then the divisions between Laibach and the rest of NSK have deepened, with Laibach launching, with the release of its 2014 album *Spectre*, a new party, also called Spectre; those who sign up are warned: 'You can't leave the Party. But the Party can leave you.'

Laibach's concert in Pyongyang a year later, the first performance in the Democratic People's Republic of Korea by a Western pop group, showed that it was still willing to mirror Stalinism as its main project, critically mirror it and over-identify with it, in order to force a choice for the audience as to what they were willing to collude with and enjoy while doing so. The bureaucrats looked dumbfounded, and the Argentinean ambassador who had his hands over his ears during the concert said that listening to the music was "like torture".

Love

One of the lessons of psychoanalysis is that the fantasy that we have freely chosen our identities is an illusion, a powerful necessary illusion charged with enjoyment, and that's why we also enjoy differentiating ourselves from others whose identities clash with ours, and that is also why we direct so much hatred at those who threaten to undermine this identity. That is what is brought alive in transference, the clinical relationship in which the construction of identity is disturbed, a relationship in which love relationships are repeated onto the figure of the analyst and where the analyst is sometimes hated for questioning where those love relationships and forms of identity have come from.

Way back in 1993, after Laibach had been demonised in Slovenia and NSK State in Time had been formed as a response to the country's independence from Yugoslavia, Žižek published an essay defending them with the suggestive title 'Why are Laibach and NSK not Fascists?' Žižek had already argued elsewhere that NSK State in Time provided a symbolic apparatus that could provide an alternative to European citizens in shock at the fragmentation of existing state institutions. The problem was not so much that archaic hatreds were always bubbling away beneath the surface in Bosnia-Herzegovina, for example, ready to explode when the veneer of civilisation was stripped away. That would be the fear of psychoanalytic commentators in thrall to an energetic, stereotypical hydraulic model of the unconscious. It is this misrepresentation of Žižek that we were treated to in Chantal Mouffe's explanation for group conflict in Yugoslavia when she visited Manchester. Instead, the civil war allowed for the expression of hatreds that had already been structurally woven into the fabric of the existing state institutions, incited by them. To propose, as NSK State did, a temporal shared identity rather than a geographically-based one was a progressive alternative.

The choice posed by Laibach, however, was of a different order, and the anxiety the band provoked in their audience was necessary if one was to avoid replacing the discourse of the master that permeates much state politics with the discourse of the university, a no less authoritarian way of educating people, inducting them into one single, totalising view of the world. Just as the Lacanian psychoanalyst works with the transference, knowing that whatever they say will be interpreted by the analysand as being a manifestation of the transference relation itself – no metalanguage can be spoken, remember – so Laibach refuse to tell their audiences what to think. To do that would fail anyway. Žižek argues that Laibach operate through a kind of transference, Lacanian psychoanalytic transference, that should never be interpreted as such by the analyst.

As the band warned twenty years after Žižek's essay, in the lyrics to 'We Are Time', 'we are not here to please you'. We shall, they intone in sinister vein, 'give you nothing. And in return, we will take even less'. This is not strictly true, of course, for they will gladly take the entrance fee to their concerts as well as the income from the tacky merchandise that those who are willing to take up the position of a 'fan' will supply them with. Just as the psychoanalyst will take a fee for their time. What is most important, however, is the symbolic charge of the transference relationship, in which the analysand will never get the love they demand from their analyst, and the analyst will never accept love back. The analysand, like the Laibach audience, must take responsibility for their own decision about what to make of what they hear, and then, in the end, let it go. They can't be told how to do that. They must do it for themselves.

I am not sure if what Laibach and NSK are doing is really an 'application' of psychoanalysis. It is not applying psychoanalysis as a theoretical framework to interpret social phenomena. The risk with that standard approach, a danger that is particularly evident in academic research, is that it simply reframes and redescribes topics in psychoanalytic language. Such academic research approaches effectively perform in the social realm what some psychoanalysts do in the clinic, which is to inject their own signifiers into the speech they hear there. Lacanian psychoanalysis in the clinic, in contrast, takes care to utilise the signifiers that appear in the analysand's speech, underlining those signifiers that repeat, punctuating the sessions in such a way as to draw attention to these signifiers without directly 'interpreting' them. There is an irony that Lacanian cultural-political theory sometimes falls into the same trap as academic research and traditional 'applied psychoanalysis' in the social realm outside the clinic. That often entails a betrayal of psychoanalysis as such.

Laibach and NSK are closer to the kind of research interventions that break from supposedly neutral, objective investigation and engage, instead, in 'action research', designed to bring about changes in the world. This is not, of course, democratic 'participatory action research' because it does not pretend to even out power relations between researcher and researched. On the contrary, Laibach and NSK accentuate those power relations; they accentuate them so that we can see more clearly how power operates and how attached we are to power. They are close to psychoanalysis insofar as they enact psychoanalysis itself in the process, bringing to life psychoanalytic concepts, and, perhaps, in this way they also provide an opportunity for noticing the limits of psychoanalysis itself.

So, with that, it is time now for us to shift focus, from attempts to 'apply' psychoanalysis while attending to its limits to discussions of psychoanalysis where the limits of the approach are foregrounded. The final four chapters are therefore concerned in different ways with the limits of psychoanalysis – in Japan, Russia, Islam and then back at the borders of the clinic.

17

JAPAN

A limit case for analysis

This chapter begins to examine the cultural-historical conditions for psychoanalysis to exist, looking at underlying assumptions about the self and others in Central and Western Europe, and describing the ways in which different versions of psychoanalysis have taken root in Japan and Korea. This throws into relief how ideas about subjectivity, which make it possible for this clinical practice to take and work, are necessarily local, limited. This examination is one way of tackling the opposition between particularity and universality.

A

A is for *amae*, which is Takeo Doi's signature concept, by means of which he claimed to have developed a specifically Japanese psychoanalytic description of child-rearing and adult relationships. Doi then claimed to have extended this notion so that it would operate as a universally-applicable discovery about the nature of human dependence on others. This curious contradictory claim for *amae* is yet another example of a continually-recurring tension within psychoanalysis; there is acknowledgement that the theoretical framework and clinical practice developed in Europe towards the end of the nineteenth century were particularly suited for that culture, and there are attempts to read psychoanalytic narratives back into history and across the world to find proof that Freud was really discovering the unconscious rather than inventing it.

Freud himself is hesitant about claiming universal validity for psychoanalysis as a scientific discovery, arguing very clearly, for example, that psychoanalysis should not be a world view; for Freud, the closest psychoanalysis comes to a world view is to the supposed world view of science, a historically-emergent mode of reasoned inquiry that succeeds animism and religion, and that even scientific methodology is not itself a world view as such. Lacan finesses this, agreeing that psychoanalysis is not scientific, but arguing that psychoanalysis operates upon the 'subject of science', that is, upon a historically-specific kind of human subject divided between experience and forms of knowledge that go beyond them. And Lacan drums this home with repeated references to Freud's 'invention' of psychoanalysis, which, I believe, we should also interpret as meaning that Freud also invented the unconscious and all the theoretical paraphernalia that fleshes out an image of the human being – one that was born with scientific reason, and sustained and elaborated under a capitalist political-economic system in which alienation is endemic.

That was my starting point for a social-constructionist research project into the nature of psychoanalysis in Japan, a project that had a faltering false start before I began my psychoanalytic training in the mid-1990s and only got going after I had finished that training, when I was able to visit Japan with Erica and meet first with Takeo Doi as the most well-known Japanese psychoanalyst in 2004. "I am very old," he said as he unwrapped his present, a framed mirror-image of nature by our friend back in Manchester, 1930s Kindertransport émigré Marion Daltrop, a social worker who used psychoanalytic ideas in her own work with disturbed children. Doi opened the present while we were there, a playful, defiant gesture that broke from the Japanese rule of etiquette, which requires that a present be politely accepted, put away, and opened after the guest has left.

Doi was, indeed, quite old. Born in 1920, Doi was shaped in his career as an analyst as much by the US occupation at the end of the Second World War as by Japanese culture, travelling to the US to train in psychiatry and psychoanalysis, absorbing the tenets of ego-psychology there, and puzzling over the difference between Japan and the US in his most well-known book, *The Anatomy of Dependence*, which was originally published in Japanese in 1971 as *Amae no Kōzō*.

Doi became a mainstay of the International Psychoanalytical Association in Japan, though, when we met him at his office in the centre of Tokyo, the Japan Psychoanalytical Society had just come out of a very rocky ride with the IPA. The IPA had discovered that its Japanese franchise had been fiddling its records to cover up the fact that instead of ensuring that trainee analysts underwent five-times-a-week psychoanalysis, they had been letting people through into membership after attending once a week. This was because of the cost and the small number of practising IPA analysts in the country.

This was most embarrassing at a time when the IPA was insisting that it was the gold standard of training, and the British Psychoanalytical Society was already busy covering up the fact that IPA analysts in one of its own organisations in France were only required to see a training analyst during their training only three times a week. I pointed this out in a contribution to the NWIDP newsletter in 2004, claiming that my colleague John Churcher, now a Manchester-based IPA analyst, the only one, had copied and pasted the misleading claim about the necessity of five-times-a-week analysis from the British Society website. He was most aggrieved, pointing out that he had written the passages himself and then they had been put in the article and on the website. But still, sorry, the claim itself was still misleading.

The Japan Psychoanalytic Society, JPS, had to apologise profusely for misleading the IPA and was now, in 2004, tightening up its training. It was clear that there was much variation in training around the world, and that the issue of the particularity of psychoanalysis in Japan was a rather sensitive one. Psychoanalysis first developed here in the 1920s, and there were very soon rival translations of Freud's writings, and some quaint innovations in the practice, with the first analysts using a deckchair in which the analysand faced away from the analyst instead of free associating on a chaise longue. Why not, I thought. I had sat in a low-slung chair in my analysis with Amelia, and I was now seeing my analysands in a small office in the speech therapy clinic in MMU. I couldn't fit a couch into the room, and so my analysands settled into a terrible fold-up, green garden chair, like a deckchair. I also experimented with analysands sitting on a low chair in my office, a rather shambolic experience for both of us I suspect.

Much of the supposed dependence of the Japanese on their elders and betters, whether in organisations or other collective bodies, was actually imported into Japan by the US during the occupation and enforced by regimes of 'Fordist' factory production. The opposition between Western 'individualist' and Eastern 'collectivist' styles of personality formation had a stronger basis in that occupation than in the depth of Asian culture, and on top of that there were social movements that transcended this colonial binary categorisation of East and West. There was a very strong trade union movement and a proliferation of left political parties, some with substantial representation in parliament, and even a long-standing Japanese anarchist tradition. Doi did notice, however, during his time in the US, that there were cultural expectations that contrasted with what he was used to at home; that he obey the invitation to 'help himself' when he went to dinner parties, for example, was something that he was most uncomfortable with. A Japanese guest does not expect to 'help themselves', but to be helped; we had Japanese visitors in Manchester who began their visit with the phrase 'thank you for looking after me', a request and an expectation.

Amae in noun form describes the state of dependence the infant has on the mother, and this then leads the infant to *amaeru* the mother, and others later in life, a call to the other to indulge them and mother them. This attempt to deny the fact of separation from the mother is manifested in a clinging dependence on others, an *amaeuruing*, which, Doi claims, pervades Japanese culture. It is certainly true that *amae* is prevalent as a description of behaviour, appearing in literature in refined form and in pop songs as something that turns each expression of desire into desperate puppy love. It is as suffocating and exasperating for the recipient as it is for those who *amaeru* to them, an apparently pathological cultural and political process. However, Doi also insists that this dependence, something that we learn from Japanese child-rearing and relationships, is a valuable corrective to the self-centred, competitive culture of the West.

According to Doi, the Japanese have learnt from *amae* what he calls the 'psychological impossibility of freedom', and this profoundly psychoanalytic lesson about the inescapable, repetitive attempts to return to one's dependence on one's first love object provides insight into really pathological cultural and political processes. This insight includes a diagnosis of the 'morass of despair and nihilism' in the West, a diagnosis in which Doi coincides with Christopher Lasch's bewailing of the 'culture of narcissism', and a rather reactionary stance with respect to radical political movements; the search for freedom in the student movement of the 1960s in Japan, for example, is seen by Doi as childish and impossible, regressive.

There is a peculiar twist here on the tragic vision of the human predicament, which is part and parcel of psychoanalysis, developed in the heart of Europe in the nineteenth century, a vision that is at one with strains of romanticism and a gothic, morbid obsession with death. Much philosophy and cultural criticism, and then Freudian psychoanalysis, revolves around what Danish philosopher Søren Kierkegaard called 'sickness unto death', and this, of course, is something that made Freud, translated into the French existentialist tradition, attractive to Lacan. We are forever divided, and every attempt to return to a supposedly Edenic state is thwarted; as we formulate what freedom would be, we are trapped all the more in the meshwork of language, in which the word is the murder of the thing. This twist in Doi's work is particularly poignant, for it reflects something of his own marginal position in Japan, while participating in the adaptation of psychoanalysis to the dominant culture of the West.

Doi was Christian, and his book *The Anatomy of Dependence* spells out the story of Christ at great length, in order to impress upon the reader the importance of dependence and obligation to others – something that is, Doi claims, the main message of Christian scripture. Christians are a tiny minority in Japan, at one time viciously persecuted, and something of the predicament of Christianity in Japan parallels the hostility to Judaism in Western culture. There is antisemitism in Japan, but Christians have also been viewed as having undue influence, a view that intensified during the US occupation. In this respect, then, Doi as a psychoanalyst was marginalised in Japan, just as Freud was in the German-speaking centre of Europe. Not exactly the same marginalisation, but analogous, perhaps homologous. This was the case for quite a few other psychoanalysts, so what we are seeing here is some kind of weird replication in Japan of the cultural process by which psychoanalysis works at the margins, with some consequent deeper insight into the pathological aspects of the dominant culture to which they were subjected. At the same time, psychoanalysis has been adapted to Western culture, with many of the traces of Freud's own Jewish heritage obscured along the way, 'Christianised' we might say: Doi, trained as a psychoanalyst in the US, reflects that Christianisation and adaptation of psychoanalysis to the dominant culture.

I sent Doi the draft manuscript of my book *Japan in Analysis: Cultures of the Unconscious*, and sought a second audience with him to discuss the book when I visited Japan again in 2007. The book included descriptions of other forms of psychoanalysis within the frame of the Japan Psychoanalytic Society and outside it. I also discussed the work of Masafumi Nakakuki, someone who identified strongly with ego-psychology, but who reframed what Doi described in child development in more classically psychoanalytic terms, as a relationship between sadism and masochism. For Nakakuki, the masochism of the Japanese was something to be analysed, not pathologised, and he was in some ways a rival of Doi, someone who had been refused membership of the JPS. He did not meet all of the requirements of membership of the organisation as an IPA franchise, and neither, he told us, did Doi. Doi was annoyed at my book manuscript, and his letter said I obviously had learned nothing from my first visit. This is something you might bear in mind as you read the account of psychoanalysis in Japan I offer you here. It is a partial, and clearly contested, account.

2

I had better luck with the Kleinians and Winnicottians in the JPS who were very helpful. They were, like Doi, very Westernised. Osamu Kitayama, for example, had been better known in Japan as a lead singer with the 'Folk Crusaders' before devoting his time to clinical work and the internal politics of the JPS. Some of his most interesting papers are on representations in Western art of mother-infant interaction, focusing on iconic Christian paintings. Again, then, there is a tension between the elaboration of culturally-specific Japanese alternatives to Freudian theory and a claim that these discoveries translate back and forth between East and West, providing universally-applicable descriptions. When I asked Kitayama how he would account for the uptake of psychoanalysis as a European theoretical framework in Japan, he countered with a good question: "Was Freud really European?"

One of the first psychoanalysts in Japan, Heisaku Kosawa, the guy with the deckchair, tried to persuade Freud that the Hindu myth of Prince Ajase might be more applicable in the East than the story of Oedipus. There are strong proto-Kleinian inflections to the early Japanese psychoanalytic readings of the so-called 'Ajase complex'. Ajase's mother, Queen Idaike, was desperate to have a child, and was told by a soothsayer that a hermit living in the woods would be reincarnated in her womb as her son, so she killed the hermit, who imposed on her a curse as he was dying, that he would kill her husband when he grew up. Frightened that this would come to pass, she tried to kill her son when he was born, and when Ajase was told about this as an adolescent he tried to kill his mother; but failed, felt guilty, and suffered from psychosomatic sores all over his body. The queen confided in the Buddha and then devoted herself to her son, who later became a good king. Reparation all round.

There are elements that scholars of *amae* would recognise here, intense dependence of the child on the mother and then of the mother upon her child, but Kosawa saw the 'most archaic sadism' in the story, oral sadism that was apparent in accounts of Ajase's rage, and, Kosawa claimed, in the infant's drive to bite the mother, the mother who is the origin of life itself. Kosawa's protégé, Keigo Okonogi, who became one of the most important diplomatic mediators between the Japanese psychoanalysts and the IPA, then emphasised the relationship between mother and son as crucial; the figure of the king disappears from the story, note. Ego-psychologist Nakakuki acknowledged that there is some kind of narcissistic battle between the son and the father in the Ajase complex, as with the Oedipus complex, and saw the outcome of the tale as indicating 'introjection and identification with the masochistic mother', in which masochism flowers into objective self-criticism and self-discipline. What would Foucault say?

Kitayama's response to the debates over the value of the Ajase complex was to turn to a more obviously Japanese folk-myth alternative to this Hindu import, and thus bypass the influence of Buddhism in Japanese culture, looking back to origin myths that are part of the infrastructure of Shintō accounts. The question that the Ajase complex poses, and that the popular story of Urashima Taro solves, according to Kitayama, is how the son escapes from the mother if the father is not there. Classical psychoanalysis would have it that the father intervenes between the child and their first love object, usually the mother, and so the father operates as a 'third term' in the Oedipal triangle of mother, infant and father. For any psychoanalyst worth their salt what is most important in the Oedipus complex is the triangle itself, not the way it is mapped onto real fathers or mothers. At root is the question as to how you escape from the first love object in order to enter culture composed of other beings in the world, whether lovers or rivals for love.

Kitayama reminds his Japanese readers that the fisher-boy Urashima marries a beautiful princess in an undersea palace who gives him a box that he should not open. Urashima carries the box home and, guess what, he does open it, suddenly becomes old and dies. He does not obey the prohibition 'don't look'. The same pattern is to be found in the founding myth of the birth of Japan in which Izanami, who has given birth to a fire god and burnt her genitals in the process, forbids her husband Izanagi to follow her into the land of the dead. He too disobeys the prohibition 'don't look', and only just escapes with his life after Izanami wreaks her revenge. In both cases, Kitayama argues, we see our hero's demand to look as 'obviously connected,' he says, 'with the oral demand towards the mother's breast which may be extended to her body to rob it of its good contents,' which is, again, pretty classical Kleinian fare.

The JPS analysts who look to Japanese myths as alternative culturally-sensitive anchor-points for a theory of the Japanese psyche, also have to fight a rearguard battle against analysts who have always been much happier in the field of myth, the Jungians. In fact the Jungians in Japan have slightly more members of their organisations than members of the IPA in Japan. They also have a powerful media profile through Hayao Kawaii, who trained in Zurich, the Mecca of analytical psychology, through his son Toshio Kawaii, and through the popular novelist Haruki Murakami, who mingles everyday encounters with cats with magical realist scenarios involving iconic Shintō, manga-like life-forms. Here it is as if the archetypes of the collective unconscious that Jung describes are brought alive, brought to the surface and confirmed for their audience as the stuff of the self.

While many of the psychoanalysts, including the Jungians, look back, some of the currents of work, among the many Western imports of new technologies of the self, compatible with the search for meaning and self-management that alienation under capitalism incites, also go with more futuristic metaphors. Group analysis exists in

Japan, for example, but its association to the key concept of the approach, the 'group matrix', is not so much linked with the maternal but with the machinic nature of contemporary society. For Foulkes, the founder of group analysis, the matrix signifies the interwoven shared reality of the group constructed by its members, and conjures up images of the mother and the womb, both 'mother' and 'womb' having etymological roots linked with 'matrix' in Latin and Middle English.

While members of group analytic forums in the West often free associate to this kind of maternal imagery, those in Japan are apparently more cued in to the streams of green flickering zeros and ones in the film *The Matrix*, an already-existing construction of reality to which we are subject, from which we cannot escape. This can also be the negative space of contemplative activity, *ma*, a different kind of 'ma' to that which is associated with the matrix in the West, one that is valued in groups in Japan, included in group analytic ones.

Z

Z is for Zen, for meditation on irresolvable contradictions at the heart of existence that leads, if not to an escape from suffering, to an acceptance of the cycle of birth and death and rebirth that is the human condition. In Zen Buddhism we can find ourselves in that 'it-ness' of our existence that we too often avoid as we try to shore up an image of the self, as if that were the centre of our lives. There is a radical rereading here of the famous phrase Freud employs in his 1933 New Introductory Lectures to describe the end of analysis, in which he says 'Where id was, there ego shall be'. At least, this is what the English translation of the lecture says. In the German original, it is '*Wo Es war, soll Ich Werden*', where it was, there I should become. The phrase is followed by a metaphorical elaboration, which does fit quite well with the common reading and English rendition, where Freud says that this is the work of culture, not unlike the draining of the Zuider Zee. It does then indeed look as if the aim of psychoanalysis is, as the ego-psychologists would have it, to strengthen the ego or the 'I' and to drain the id or the 'it' as if it were a dangerous swamp.

However, if we are to obey the precepts of Zen Buddhism, we should surely try to lose the self, dissolve the ego, rather than buttress it; just such an argument is made by Erich Fromm, for example, who is critical of the acquisitive mode of 'having' in capitalist society and looks instead to a broader, more generous sense of 'being'. It is that sense of ourselves in something bigger, of our nature and of a universe we cannot control, that psychoanalysis leads us towards. We should not aim to pit ourselves against the unconscious, but discover ourselves there. It is also in that reading of Freud's phrase that Jacques Lacan pits himself against ego-psychology. When we asked the Kyoto-based Lacanian psychoanalyst Kazushige Shingu what the difference was between psychoanalysis and Japanese Buddhism, he replied that there really is no difference if it really is psychoanalysis.

Shingu, who has been part of an ambitious project retranslating all of Freud's writings, taking responsibility for *The Interpretation of Dreams*, mines the connections between Japanese Buddhism and Lacan. Shingu is a serene master; we addressed him in public events as Shingu Sensei, Master Shingu, and also, note, he still practises as a psychiatrist, dispensing diagnoses and medication. His reinterpretation of Sophocles' play *Antigone*, for example, relates the motif of 'between two deaths', which Lacan makes big play with in his Seminar VII on ethics, to Buddhist acceptance of our mortality. Antigone is walled up in her brother's tomb to suffer a physical death from starvation, subject also to the 'second death' in which she will be erased from the symbolic, completely forgotten. Shingu points out that while Buddhism in Japan often consoles its adepts with the soothing idea that there will be a time of judgement and a hope for 'Nirvana' after they have died, after they have been subject to the first death, one of the lessons of psychoanalysis is actually in line with the more authentic and painful thought that there will be what is referred to in Japanese Buddhism as 'the other death'. Psychoanalytic practice in tune with Japanese culture would, then, enable the subject to give up on the big Other, to give up on the idea that there is escape from the second death, and be ready to anticipate and accept the second death, erasure from the symbolic, while they are still physically alive. Tell that to modern subjects on Facebook. Beyond the pleasure principle is death, not, as first translations into Japanese had it, 'the other shore of enjoyment'.

Japan is often treated as a 'limit case' for Western accounts of subjectivity, including psychoanalytic accounts, with Japanese culture seen as most inscrutably 'Other' to the West. This is why so much cross-cultural research in psychology and sociology obsessively worries away at the differences between the West and Japan as two cultures that have taken parallel paths toward modernisation and a capitalist economy. In fact, despite the attempts to insulate Japan from the outside world during the Edo period – from the beginning of the seventeenth century to the middle of the nineteenth – Japan has undergone rapid industrialisation heavily influenced by the West, by US occupation, and then by an active enthusiastic absorption back into its culture of foreign images of Japan. A popular genre of literary and social-scientific writing is *Nihonjinron*, that is, theories and discussions about the Japanese, and this also feeds each and every variety of psychoanalysis that encounters another culture to itself, that speculates about what is different about it, and then finds itself incorporated into Japan.

We were repeatedly told that there was some kind of mirror-image 'twinship' between England and Japan, two island kingdoms in which the inhabitants share the same concern with politesse, a reserve toward foreigners and, if the speaker was more liberal, even some acknowledgement of unfortunate legacies of imperial power exercised upon other nations. We noticed this most powerfully when we crossed on the Beetle Ferry from Hakata to Busan in South Korea, transported in the space of three hours from a quiet, ordered world to noisy, chaotic bustle. This kind of atmosphere, if it were to be found in Japan, would be expected in the small Brazilian community and among returnees from the very large Japanese community in São Paulo: Brazilians have a reputation among the Japanese for being noisy, disruptive of '*ma*'.

There is much discussion among Korean psychoanalysts about their relationship with Confucianism – a prescription for social order in which you must learn to defer to the good sense of your elders and betters – but the Korean Lacanians we spoke to in the capital, Seoul, were among the liveliest, most effervescent, outgoing bunch we have ever met. If Japan is like England, then Korea, which was once occupied by Japan, is, we were told, like Ireland, England's oldest colony. Many of the academics we encountered were working on psychoanalysis and Irish literature, on Joyce, about whom Lacan wrote in Seminar XXIII, on the sinthome, and on Beckett, who was analysed by Bion; "We are the Irish of the East," one of them said, as if that explained it. Just as Christians in Japan are a minority faith, implicitly linked with psychoanalysis because practitioners have personal links with that faith, so in Korea it is specifically Catholics who are a sizeable minority population with access to education, including to psychoanalytic academic training.

We kneeled politely at a low table in a Korean restaurant, and were asked in a playfully mocking way whether we thought we were in Japan; the other customers were lounging around with their legs splayed about. Discussion after lectures at the Korean Society for Lacan and Contemporary Psychoanalysis was robust. During one question time I was told via a translator that an audience member had said that my answer was unsatisfactory and I should say some more. Then we were taken for late-night chicken and chips and they all got very drunk, laughing as they explained who had what official role in their psychoanalytic society, as if it were a ridiculous pantomimic charade. They staggered out of the bar and stood in a line on the pavement to wave us off when we took a taxi back to our hotel.

English psychoanalysts, it should be said, are, as a rule, very English, and calculated reserve inside the clinic often extends to po-faced refusal to engage in small talk with colleagues outside it. Something of that was what was going on, I guess, in the CFAR training sessions, where the trainees were cautiously trying to work out what the rules of appropriate behaviour were in a new subculture they were anxious to prove themselves to be part of. It is so very different in Dublin, where the Lacanians there are more like the Koreans. I accompanied Kazushige Shingu from Kyoto and Chris Dunker from São Paulo to give some talks in Dublin in 2006; in the evening Chris found an old football and kicked it across to the startled figure we usually referred to as Shingu Sensei shouting "Come on Kaz, let's play a game!". The Brazilian breaks 'ma'.

Lacan commented once that the Japanese were 'unanalysable', but then he said the same about Catholics. Maybe the open secret of psychoanalysis is that we all are, that psychoanalysis as something 'interminable', as Freud put it, is impossible. Attempts to implant psychoanalysis in another culture miss the point. It won't work there because it won't work at home, wherever that is.

18

QUEER

From Russia with love

More limits. In this chapter I expand the scope of this study of psychoanalysis and its limits to describe some contemporary debates and tensions inside theory and practice over the role of the family, gender and sexuality. I do this by describing recent connections between psychoanalysis and queer theory, visiting Russia to see how it works out there. We will need to take a little journey through queer, however, before we arrive in Russia. We will get there eventually. Bear with me.

Discourse

I first heard the word 'queer' as a positive performative twisting of gender and sexuality at the first Discursive Construction of Knowledge conference in Adelaide in February 1994. Why 'performative'? I knew of Queer Nation, an activist group founded by members of ACT-UP in New York fighting for lesbian and gay rights, and, crucially, fighting for increased production and distribution of antiretroviral drugs for HIV/AIDS. Michel Foucault had died of AIDS in 1984, the virus named as HIV two years later, and in 1990, when Queer Nation was formed, Judith Butler had just published her path-breaking book *Gender Trouble*, following that up in 1993 with *Bodies that Matter*. Her second book responded to criticism that her real 'queer' book, which was the book that made her one of the patron saints of queer politics, had reduced sex as well as gender to discourse.

Žižek made the nasty, rather jealous, sideswipe when I met him ten years later, that those two books should have been titled 'Body Trouble' and 'Gender that Matters', the point being, I guess, that Butler had indeed dissolved bodies into discourse and then reduced matter to gender politics. He didn't like feminists, and I guessed that he didn't like lesbians. Butler was also Jewish, and I eventually had to transcribe most of the interviews I had conducted in 2003 myself; a Jewish research assistant at MMU commented "he doesn't like Jews" after a couple of hours of work on the tapes, and obviously felt uncomfortable. I defended him. Žižek referred to his three-way debate with Butler and Laclau in *Contingency, Hegemony, Universality* as "my orgy book".

Butler was a good deal cannier than that, however, and the whole point of her critique, and inspiration to queer 'third-wave' feminist activists, revolved around the subversion of the relationship between gender and sexuality, such that gender was seen as constituted by the 'performative' naming of boys and girls. The performance of gender was not seen as conscious play-acting, even though gender identities did come to be seen as central to the ego, but as the non-conscious repetition of categories of gender that then laid down the matrix for sexual identification and sexual desire. One consequence of that performative dimension of gender and sexuality was that the 'queering' of those categories was also a queering of identity as such, even if the terms 'lesbian' and 'gay' might still be re-enacted tactically in order to construct alliances of the oppressed with 'men' and 'women'. All men and women are, if we take psychoanalysis seriously, already queer. Steven Angelides at the Adelaide conference insisted that 'queer' was a verb not a noun, and if it ever became crystallised as a kind of identity so that activists would declare themselves as queer, "then," Steven said, "we'll drop the term and move on, find a better term that stays with what we are doing."

Fast forward fifteen years and there was a lot of queer theory and queer politics around, even queer identity, with activists working at the boundaries of academia. The term was also beginning to appear as a flag of convenience in psychoanalytic debate. It was continuing to serve well in the radical letter-string LGBT, even if some of these folk, as well as some straight allies, were identifying as queer, and that letter-string was still proliferating at an alarming rate, in a way that was sometimes disconnected from politics, in academic debate. So when two Irish analysts, Eve Watson, a Lacanian, and Noreen Giffney, a Kleinian, asked me to write a commentary on six queer theoretical papers for a book they were assembling, to write as a psychoanalyst, I jumped at the chance. This might be a chance not only to bridge the two domains, to really queer psychoanalysis, but also to link clinical practice with psychoanalytic theory. The plan was that after the commentaries there would be a third layer of chapters that would reflect on the intersections that had been created. This would take a while to follow through.

The chapters arrived in the post in 2010, a weird collection of papers in which it seemed that the authors had already achieved for queer theory what Freud had taken such pains to warn psychoanalysis against. No, psychoanalysis is not a world view, nor should it aim to become one, Freud insisted, but now most of these queer theorists elaborated in startlingly exhaustive ways how their approach not only expressed something of their own attachment to the signifier 'queer' but served as an all-encompassing frame through which to view the world and their place in it. We were told, for example, that Winnicott was queer, did he but know it, that the love of dogs was queer, did they but know it, better not, and even that the love of God was queer.

There were, you might guess, some stabs at links with psychoanalysis in some of the papers, but these were scattered and contradictory. There was no necessary problem with that, and although my task was to write something Lacanian, I was not going to pretend that Lacan was queer or that you needed to go to a Lacanian psychoanalyst if you thought you were or thought you wanted to be queer. After all, Saint Judith was herself in analysis with an IPA analyst, and she plucked what she wanted from the history of psychoanalysis, queering this and that, and using psychoanalytic theory to give her own theoretical interventions another twist.

'Queer' sure was a signifier, and Lacan, he say that a signifier represents a subject for another signifier. That is what is going on in the four discourses, for example: the subject as such is never actually a subject as such, but is always defined by the gap and movement between signifiers. This is a gap and movement that is difficult to capture in written form, and the kind of theoretical writing that tries to spell out what 'queer' really is always risks falling into the trap of pinning down and defining what is appearing moment by moment in discourse as the unconscious opens and closes. The only way to break through that alienated empty speech, which always situates the subject as a subject of the statement, is to speak, to open the way to the subject of the enunciation, to enable the enunciating subject to appear in their speech. Even then, in the clinic, it is very likely that this truth only appears at those moments to the speaking subject, not to the psychoanalyst who must put the speech in a grid if they want to convey something intelligible about what is happening in the clinic to their colleagues in clinical case presentations or in books about psychoanalysis.

One question was whether queer opened things up or closed them down. It would close them down if it functioned as a kind of postmodern version of evenly suspended attention to a variety of different theories and practices of subjectivity. That is, if it loosens its hold on reality such that it has no stake in it, as if every story we tell about ourselves were equivalent; if that were the case then the kind of therapy that would be most fitting for queer sensibility would be a narrative or discursive or postmodern constructionist approach that was completely agnostic about the unconscious. There was a risk queer would operate in that way if it followed in the tracks of those who made academic careers out of it as a 'theory'.

It would open things up, however, if queer functioned as it had done in political activism, which attended to power, to the way that power relations and identity categories were performatively unconsciously reiterated. We do not know exactly what we do, and psychoanalysis is not about what we think about but what we repeat, whether we think about it or not. And transference in the clinic is precisely about power: the way to tackle it is not to pretend that it does not exist, but to work through how relations of power are reiterated, performed in the clinic in the transference.

Matter

We are almost in Russia now. I know it is a long journey, but a necessary one. The queer psychoanalysis book was still waiting for its third-level commentaries in 2013, for commentaries that should not, of course, pretend to provide a 'meta-narrative' or, in Lacanian terms, a metalanguage that would explain what the encounter between the queer theorists and the psychoanalysts was really about. There is no comprehensive world view, and no metalanguage that successfully sums things up. We know this from the clinic where every interpretation, however carefully we spell things out, will be heard in the transference as coming from a particular position that the analysand has already constructed, as they conjure into place a particular kind of subject to whom they are speaking, speaking to what Lacan calls the 'subject supposed to know'.

I was invited to Russia, and, even better than that, so was David Pavón Cuéllar. In 2006 he had sent me a copy of his book *Le révolutio-m'être* from Rouen in France. The book, the enigmatic title of which translates very roughly among its different ambiguous semiotic permutations as something like 'I am the revolution', 'applied' elements of Lacan's theory of discourse to a very brief extract from an interview with a leader of the Ejército Popular Revolucionario, a guerrilla group in Mexico. I wanted this book to be in English as soon as I saw it, for David Pavón Cuéllar was clearly using this application of Lacanian discourse theory to a short piece of text in order to explicate better what 'Lacanian discourse theory' was. I met David, an impressive activist and academic, and then managed to persuade Karnac Books, a psychoanalytic publisher in London, to take on the book in a new list called 'Lines of the Symbolic'. It was published in 2010 as *From the Conscious Interior to an Exterior Unconscious: Lacan, Discourse Analysis and Social Psychology*, a book that David rewrote in the process in order to key into English-language debates about discourse and psychoanalysis in what was emerging as 'psychosocial studies'. The second book in the series, which appeared a year later, was Chris Dunker's historical masterwork *The Structure and Constitution of the Psychoanalytic Clinic*, which, in its Portuguese-language edition, was published in Brazil as *Estrutura e constituição da clínica psicanalítica: Uma arqueologia das práticas de cura psicoterapi e tratamento* and won the prestigious Prêmio Jabuti literary award.

There were already fierce 'psychosocial' debates between Kleinians and Lacanians, and between psychoanalytic psychosocial researchers and those who wanted to use other frameworks, such as those they extracted from the work of Gilles Deleuze. Those debates sometimes revolved around the use of a hyphen to signify that you were Kleinian, 'psycho-social', against the Lacanian psychosocial people who were caricatured as wanting to dissolve everything into discourse, the same kind of specious charge that had long been made against queer theory. David Pavón Cuéllar's book was the first, and still is the best, account of a Lacanian discursive framework for analysing texts. Together, we also set to work on a lengthy project for an edited book on Lacanian discourse analysis, in which we focused on what we called 'textual indeterminacy', ruptures in discourse: these would be ruptures of the Real that cut through the illusory, imaginary understanding that speakers and writers and researchers had of the meaning of texts and the symbolic frames that defined horizons of meaning as if they were fixed and deterministic. David got some money from a Mexican grant foundation for the project and we managed to get the book published almost simultaneously in Spanish and English in 2013 as *Lacan, Discourse, Event.*

Working with David Pavón Cuéllar on this Lacanian discourse project, and visiting Morelia in Mexico where he was based, opened up another panorama of psychoanalytic work. This was a context in which there were still existing schools of Frommian psychoanalysts, and, of course, Lacanians of different stripes, among whom was the Argentinian émigré Néstor Braunstein. Many of the Mexican psychoanalysts were also of the left, so David was able to recruit some of them to contribute to our book, not as easy a task as it might seem because it meant tracing delicate paths through minefields of dissension over Lacanian theory as well as Marxist politics. David and I were on the last stretch of the Lacanian discourse project when we were invited to Russia, to a conference in December 2013 on 'Psychoanalytic Discourse and Contemporary Society', which would be held in Izhevsk, capital of the Udmurt Republic, about a thousand kilometres east of Moscow. My son Adam was up for the trip. Erica was also invited, but thought it was a stupid idea to go at that time of the year when it would be freezing cold. It was.

We met David in Moscow. He arrived at the hotel in the early morning, a delayed flight, just in time for us to get a flight together to Kazan, capital of Tatarstan, where Alexander Luria, the renowned neuroscientist had been born and had founded the Kazan Psychoanalysis Study Group in 1922. Tatarstan has a Muslim-majority population and Kazan has many mosques, one of which is inside the local Kremlin, the fortress administrative complex for the city. Lenin had been expelled from Kazan University in 1887, and so we also trekked around in the deep icy snow to find his house and the lecture room in the university where he sat when he was studying. We had bought a SIM card in Moscow and followed texted instructions to collect our train tickets in Kazan, and then, guided by regular texts from Maria Melnikova in Izhevsk, took the five-hour trip to Agryz, where we were met by Dimitry Grebenkin and driven through the glowing white night landscape to Izhevsk.

The first day of the conference had been in Russian. We arrived in time for the second day, with temporary permits to enter Udmurt State University. Our visas, eventually, after many tortuous negotiations over who had the authority to issue official letters of invitation to the conference, had to be tourist only, something that could have been problematic in getting to Izhevsk, which was closed to foreigners when it was in the Soviet Union because of its armaments industry. On the second day of the conference I gave my paper on 'Queer Developments in Psychoanalysis'. The argument of my paper, which was painfully translated sentence-by-sentence into Russian as I watched the blank-faced audience try to make sense of it, was that authentic psychoanalysis was always, already, itself 'queer'. The argument was as follows.

Freud argued that human beings are 'constitutionally bisexual', and so adult relationships are moulded by experiences of first love objects, which are accorded characteristics of gender and sexual orientation on the basis of dominant social norms. The first designation of the infant as being a boy or a girl sets in play a series of assumptions about what kind of sexual being the child will be and what kind of sex they will want as an adult. In Lacanian terms, we can conceptualise how the first relationships with an image of the other, which becomes one of the templates for the ego in the mirror-stage, are then re-signified and reordered as the child learns to speak. At that point the child enters the Symbolic order and the Symbolic order also enters them as the unconscious, constituted as, Lacan says, the discourse of the Other.

There is also a crucial point here about the dialectical interrelationship between the mirror-stage imaginary processes, processes that lay down the coordinates of identity in the nascent ego, and the symbolic naming of what that child is like and what it wants. It is tempting to think of the Imaginary as prior to the Symbolic, as if there is a straight developmental line linking one to the other, but Lacan subtly, but significantly, rewrote his account of the mirror-stage, for a paper given at the fourteenth IPA congress at Marienbad in 1936. The published version from 1949 clearly indicates that the framing of the imaginary relationship between infant and mother is already symbolic. The question of what a child is and what a mother is, and how they are expected to relate to each other, is a cultural-historical matter. Each is implicated in a series of 'performative' activities, the meaning of which goes well beyond them, the conditions of possibility for which precede and exceed them. You don't need Deleuze and Guattari to tell you that there is a problem when this psychoanalytic account is then 'familialised'.

Freud is also very clear that the infant is, he says, 'polymorphously perverse'; that is, the infant gets sexual gratification from each and every erogenous zone, and, in fact, from other parts of the body too. The very notion of what is 'sexual' is not yet divided off and localised in specific organs, in the genitals. It is more accurate, Freud suggests, to speak of this infantile sexuality as being a sensual experience in which bodily pleasure becomes tied to specific kinds of activity, including feeding, and so also to specific kinds of object, to those who are the primary caregivers. The restriction of this sensuality to the genitals and the construction of a particular kind of fantasised link to significant others is what gives rise to what we call 'sex'. When psychoanalysts say that infants are sexual beings, and that sexual fantasies are operative from a very early age, they do not mean that infants are like adults. That is an adult fantasy about the child. Instead, Freud draws attention to the infantile sensuality that many adults disavow and that they may reconnect with in psychoanalysis.

In the clinic, then, we make no assumptions about what is 'normal' or 'abnormal' in sexual choice, exploring *how* those choices have been made instead of moralising about which would have been the right path to follow. We 'queer' sexuality in the clinic, putting into question the heterosexual choices made by analysands just as we do any other such strange sexual proclivity. Psychoanalysis is queer, and the clinic is a queer space.

I finished. There was silence, and since the to-and-fro with the translation had taken so much time, there were no questions. It would, of course, in the Udmurt Republic, as with anywhere else in Russia, have been courting danger to ask a question that appeared to publicly legitimise homosexuality. Formal legal rights had been no protection against prohibition levelled against what the Putin regime called lesbian and gay 'propaganda', and Russian Orthodox and neo-fascist activists had physically attacked gays on the streets. In the break after my paper some people, those who could speak English, came up to me to say they liked what I said and they talked about the homophobic political atmosphere, and the difficulties this posed for psychoanalysis. I was told that many of the blank faces in the audience may have been because throughout my paper the term 'queer' had been translated as 'strange'. Psychoanalysis as strange psychoanalysis, well I suppose it was, it is.

Later in the day there were some Skype-link presentations. Carol Owens, a Lacanian from Dublin, talked about *Breaking Bad*, and Alain Vanier from Paris told us why Lacan was right about Marx, and why Marx was wrong. That was a familiar argument. David Pavón Cuéllar then talked about Lacan and Lenin, a stunning paper that revolved around the question of how the Russian Revolution as an 'event' had a peculiar relationship with time. Lenin's calculations over the correct moment at which to mobilise so that the working class, under the leadership of the Bolshevik Party, could seize power were read through Lacan and the Lacanian philosopher Alain Badiou, a figure who had loomed large in our co-edited *Lacan, Discourse, Event* book. Curiously and encouragingly, David's paper, in contrast to mine on queer, was enthusiastically received, with many questions and much discussion from students at the conference. I wished I had talked about Lenin too.

Dialectics

After the conference we celebrated the Russian translation of my *Psychoanalytic Culture* book, published by ERGO, the publishing house the psychoanalytic group ran in Izhevsk, and on the following days visited the Kalashnikov factory and the archives of the Russian Psychoanalytical Society. ERGO had already translated my book on Žižek and published many other papers by me in their journal *Anthropopraxis* and their *Annual* of psychoanalysis, including the long essay that appears at the end of my 2009 book *Psychoanalytic Mythologies*. Sergey Sirotkin, who headed the group at Udmurt State University and who is director of the ERGO publishing house, had, along with Dimitry, visited Manchester over twenty years before, and I had had some contact with them via a PhD student who worked with them later on a drug addiction project. Then, with easier email contact, they devoted more time to psychoanalysis and asked me for things they could translate. Maria, who had managed our progress from Moscow via Kazan to Izhevsk, I met for the first time, and she showed me pictures of her cats on her phone. The fourth key figure in the group was Irina Chirkova who is a manager at ERGO.

The archives were in Sergey Sirotkin's office in cardboard boxes on a shelf adjacent to a large poster of Freud. In one folder there was an application letter from the socio-cultural child researcher Lev Vygotsky to join the Society in 1925, and in another there were minutes of meetings taken by neuropsychologist Alexander Luria. I took out of another folder a handwritten note from 1930, a time when psychoanalysis was starting to fall out of favour after Stalin assumed power, when it was beginning to be associated with bourgeois degenerate ideas about sexuality, even with first hints of antisemitic suspicions that it was a 'Jewish science', paralleling the accusations made against it by the Nazis. By this time Izhevsk had become one of the last remaining psychoanalytic centres in the Soviet Union, far enough from Moscow to be no longer considered a threat.

We were told that Vera Schmidt, who had been a key figure in the psychoanalytic kindergarten movement in Moscow, had moved the archives to Izhevsk before she died. I asked if she was Jewish. Sergey thought she was. I asked if most of the figures involved in the Russian psychoanalytical movement were Jewish, and there was a silence before he said that, yes, possibly that was the case. The frayed handwritten note I held in my hand was a short message to the Society saying that because they had not been participating they should now be considered as retired from the Society, signed by Luria and Vygotsky, both Jews.

We were taken to Votkinsk, where Tchaikovsky was born, and we visited his house on the edge of Swan Lake; the guide told us that the composer had some 'marriage difficulties', but his homosexuality was never mentioned. In Votkinsk I also tried to explain to a group of students what the main argument of the book *Psychoanalytic Culture* was, that psychoanalytic ideas about the ego and the id and the unconscious and the meaning of dreams and slips of the tongue had, whether they were true or not, entered into popular consciousness. The students looked sceptical, and I couldn't be sure that what I noticed in English-speaking culture really did apply here. They seemed happier when I emphasised that I was interested in psychoanalysis as a set of stories we told about ourselves, and that if we knew they were stories we could then be in a better position to believe them or not. Here I was skating closer to the more liberal, postmodern version of queer, in which anything goes rather than staying true to the unconscious as Real.

Psychoanalysis had been a reference point in Russia for some of the leading Bolsheviks, and Wilhelm Reich had visited experimental schools in the 1920s, hopeful that the revolution had also re-energised the sexual lives of a population oppressed and repressed under Tsarism. The genetic epistemologist Jean Piaget, who had trained as a psychoanalyst, also visited to work with Sabina Spielrein – a patient of Jung's who had then been Piaget's analyst – murdered by the Nazis in Rostov-on-Don in 1942. Lenin himself had been rather suspicious of psychoanalysis, but Trotsky had championed it, arguing that it was one valuable approach, alongside Pavlov's behaviourist experiments, looking down into the murky depths of the psyche, and, when he was sent into exile in Turkey, Trotsky sent his daughter Zina to a psychoanalyst in Berlin.

There is a complicated history of psychoanalysis in Russia that is interwoven with attempts to make it politically acceptable, to adapt it to Russian culture, and this produced a series of intriguing paradoxes when psychoanalysis began to intersect with Marxism. Marxism as a historical materialist critique of political economy should also operate as a dialectical critique of subjectivity under capitalism, unravelling the way that forms of alienated experience are produced and showing how the forces of repression also operate much as the dreamwork does. Many of our dreams of revolt and of a world free of exploitation are symptomatic of the kind of society in which we can only dream of such things. The aim of Marxism is not so much to awaken the starvelings from their slumbers so that they can see reality exactly as it is, as to mobilise them to begin to construct history on their own terms. Marxism is as little concerned with the fixed identities of the bourgeoisie and the proletariat as psychoanalysis is with fixing things so that men can be men and women can be women. Perhaps one of the lessons of the third-wave feminist movement inspired by Judith Butler, among others, is that Marxism could and should be as queer as psychoanalysis.

'Queer Developments in Psychoanalysis' is, understandably, the only paper I have given to the ERGO group in Izhevsk that has not been translated by them and published in their journal *Anthropopraxis*, and communication with them has been sparse since the four of them, Irina, Maria, Dimitry and Sergey, waved us off at Izhevsk airport for our flight back to Moscow. The plane was ex-Aeroflot, and we walked up into the cabin from underneath it as if we were entering the belly of a cargo plane. David was already anxious about the flight, and more so when bits of the plane fell off as we trundled up the runway.

I was worried as we made our anxious journey back to Moscow that perhaps I had pushed our new friends too far with the queer argument. Since then the ERGO team have been pouring their energy into translating all of Freud's psychoanalytic writings into Russian, in increasingly difficult political-economic conditions. The Izhevsk researchers have through the years succeeded in breaking the isolation of Russian psychoanalysts, and keeping that tradition of work alive. Writing this account of the visit was an opportunity to be in contact with them again after too long an interval, and they quickly replied with friendly responses to the book manuscript, with love.

19

ISLAM

Faith in Freud

We are now travelling back to the Western world, a world that is increasingly inhabited by otherness, by the presence of other cultures experienced by so many as alien, but no more alien than could be the unconscious. Psychoanalysis voices the alienation that capitalist society creates as a condition for being a human subject, good, but it is also recuperated, neutralised and absorbed into the kind of culture that likes its belief systems to function as world views. In this chapter we home in on one particular manifestation of psychoanalysis as a world view, its commitment to secular democracy and scientific reason. We explore the role of Judaism and antisemitism in the history of psychoanalysis, of its place in Christian culture, and of attempts to acknowledge the impact of a 'third wave' of challenge and cultural adaptation, to Islam. But, a warning, we will again have to go round the houses to get a sense of the surrounding ideological territory before we get there.

Otherness

Psychoanalysis is about otherness, the otherness of the human subject to itself that Freud specifies as lying in the nature of the unconscious, in the existence of some other realm within and beyond us, which speaks through us, and over which we will never have full control. Free association is the 'fundamental technical rule' of psychoanalytic treatment, not because we expect the analysand to say everything; precisely the reverse, it is because the speaking subject cannot say everything, and it is where they hesitate and stumble, prevaricate and slip that they reveal something of the architecture of the self, their ego. This otherness is displaced and projected onto specific others in forms of racism, and sometimes it is also idealised in forms of mystical experience, which become sedimented in religious belief systems and institutions.

One of Freud's favourite jokes was the caption from a newspaper cartoon in the 1880s that showed a lion waiting for lunch and yawning; the caption was 'twelve o'clock and no negro'. Freud used to repeat this phrase when a patient failed to turn up for a session on time. It is hardly surprising that racism should find its way into psychoanalysis, so woven into the history of colonialism was the culture of self-reflection that emerged from the European Enlightenment. To refer to femininity as a 'dark continent', as Freud does, for example – and he writes the phrase in English, marking it while distancing himself from its many implications – illustrates how this racism is bound up with a series of oppositions in which civilisation is set against barbarism, masculinity is set against femininity, and, at root, as Lévi-Strauss argued, culture is set against nature. Frantz Fanon's analysis, again, was more necessary than ever, now being developed as anti-racist and feminist critique by Erica Burman.

This otherness also structures the way that Jews were positioned in relation to European culture at the end of the nineteenth century, the way that Freud struggled with this marginalisation and the way that psychoanalysis itself repeats it. Sander Gilman in his 1991 book *The Jew's Body* explores the way that sexuality in middle Europe, at the end of the nineteenth century, was tied to antisemitic images of degeneration and sensuality, so that the clitoris, for example, would be referred to as 'the little Jew'. Freud's own emphasis on sexuality as other to ourselves then participates in a series of semiotic links in which something of that otherness is reclaimed and something of it is still kept at bay. On the one hand we should come to be where it, the otherness, was. On the other hand, we should be reasoned enough to know what it is we are getting ourselves into.

One of the subtexts of Freud's carefully balanced appraisal of the development of reason in the West, the progressive shift from animism through to religious belief and then to scientific examination, is a rebuttal of the accusation that psychoanalysis is a 'Jewish science'. Responses to this deadly accusation have often mirrored it, and have revolved around an attempt to affirm the scientific status of psychoanalysis, on the one hand, while also acknowledging the influence of Jewish culture on the development of the practice. Freud was quite open about his identification with Hannibal who marched on Rome and nearly succeeded in defeating it, for example; and Freud then ruminates over the reasons why he might himself, as a Jew, have found it difficult to make his own journey to Rome. The famous incident in which Freud's father fails to confront an antisemite who knocks his hat off is but one of many indications that Freud was affected by this virulent pervasive form of racism from a very early age.

Acknowledging the importance of Jewish culture as a resource to be defended, even if it also means differentiating the cultured, assimilated Jews Freud himself identified with from the *Ostjuden*, the less civilised Jews from Eastern Europe, is one thing. It is trickier to acknowledge the influence of Jewish religion, something that Freud was not so keen on, though there have been attempts to link the Jewish mystical tradition and psychoanalytic practice. Kabbalistic concern with the meanings of symbols, including letters and numbers, can be detected in Freud's decomposition of dream texts into their component parts, and the nature of psychoanalytic training itself as a craft based on oral tradition and the reinterpretation of classical texts is further evidence of the influence of elements of Judaism. Perhaps it would even be possible to characterise the first wave of psychoanalytic theory and practice as operating as a form of secularised Judaism.

Psychoanalytic training is still, I discovered in CFAR, composed of theoretical discussion that revolves around the careful rereading of canonical texts; and Lacan's 'return to Freud' is a return to the meaning of Freud through such rereading, with many of his seminars dedicated to such reinterpretation. The history of psychoanalysis as such is a history of the rereadings and the tracing of debates that have taken place around those readings, which are similar to rabbinical tussles over the meaning of key religious texts. The practical training still relied on a 'transmission' of technique that was in oral form – and the translation of that into formalised bureaucratic and academic specifications of what a psychoanalyst should do in the clinic is always, necessarily, a betrayal of psychoanalysis. Enunciation is turned into statement.

Sameness

One of the most shocking aspects of the second volume of Elisabeth Roudinesco's history of psychoanalysis in France, translated into English and published by Free Association Books in 1990 as *Jacques Lacan & Co.*, is Jeffrey Mehlman's Translator's Foreword, in which Mehlman draws attention to French nationalist and antisemitic motifs in Lacan's career and writing. I had always avoided Jung for precisely this reason, suspecting that there was a deep compatibility between that pastor's son's spiritual inclinations and his racism, between speculation about archetypes of the collective unconscious and antisemitism. In this Foreword, Mehlman points out that Lacan not only comes at psychoanalysis from a French psychiatric tradition, but also from involvement in the extreme right-wing group Action Française, which was headed by the grammarian Éduard Pichon, a psychoanalyst who was president of the Societé psychanalytique de Paris from 1935 to 1937.

Lacan's progress in his own training to become a member of the SPP in 1938, when he promised to stay in analysis with Rudolf Loewenstein, remember, and then reneged on his promise, was very reluctantly agreed to by Loewenstein because there was a trade-off brokered by Pichon for Lacan, his protégé, a trade-off between Lacan's promotion and membership also being offered to Heinz Hartmann, fleeing from the Nazis. Both Loewenstein and Hartmann, along with Ernst Kris, eventually moved to the United States where they became known as the founders of ego-psychology, a current of work Lacan mercilessly criticised, including lampooning Kris as the stupid analyst of the patient who goes looking for 'fresh brains' to eat after his sessions, acting out as a message to the analyst.

Lacan's spiteful sideswipes against the IPA often slide from criticism of the adaptation of the émigrés in the United States to capitalist culture to characterisation of the analysts themselves as in some way complicit with commerce, an antisemitic trope; his claim that no Jewish psychoanalysts perished in the Nazi death camps is not only patently untrue but rings alarm bells, such statements would today be called racist dog-whistling. Lacan's manifesto statement of his own distinctive approach to psychoanalysis, in striking contrast to Freud's difficulty in journeying to Rome, is then known as the Rome discourse.

Roudinesco and Mehlman are both keen to insist that Lacan is not antisemitic. Lacan's references to his 'excommunication' from the IPA clearly signal some identification with Baruch Spinoza, excluded by the Jewish community in Amsterdam for heresy. Roudinesco defends Lacan on the basis that he was nasty about everyone, so that's settled that, it seems – but this is really beside the point. The flip side of the repeated attempts to distance himself from the Jewish heritage of psychoanalysis, is that Lacan effectively, if not deliberately, colludes in what his one-time ally André Green called the 'Christianising' of psychoanalysis. Spinoza converted to Christianity. There are implications here for the supposed 'subversive' role that Lacanian psychoanalysis plays in relation to the dominant culture. This was another disturbing aspect of the history of psychoanalysis that is sometimes simply referred to as 'The Roudinesco'; we were advised to read it, one of the few recommendations for further reading in the first meetings of my CFAR training, even though we were warned by Darian Leader that "there are some factual inaccuracies". He didn't tell us what they were.

I had assumed that Lacan's was the edgier, more radical version of psychoanalysis, but it seemed that he was very desperate to seek approval from the authorities, whether that was from the leader of the French Communist Party, to whom he sent his *Écrits*, or the Pope, with whom he sought an audience. I puzzled over what 'big Other' Lacan was writing for, and where that left psychoanalysts who were on the left. Žižek is fond of repeating Lacan's own statement that he was 'not a man of the left', and rubbing that into the faces of those who too quickly assume that Lacan is repeating the move made by first-generation psychoanalysts like Wilhelm Reich and Erich Fromm, to attempt to link psychoanalysis and Marxism. He is not. There is actually precious little of what Yannis Stavrakakis, now NSK citizen, calls in the title of his book on the topic *The Lacanian Left*. Psychoanalysis is not a leftist world view. At the same time, neither should Marxism be a world view, even though it is treated as such by those who turned it into the religion of the apparatus in the Stalinist states. It is not so easy to preserve psychoanalysis, to keep it untainted by dominant ideological practices.

It is clear from The Roudinesco that it was particularly difficult to steer clear of religion in France where there is a dominant secular tradition that is often, by default, Christian. A surprising number of founding fathers of Lacan's own school of psychoanalysis, the École freudienne de Paris, founded in 1964 after his 'excommunication' from the IPA, were Jesuit priests. Two psychoanalysts were excluded by the IPA in 1963, refused the right to train analysts. One was Lacan, and the other was Françoise Dolto, a practising Catholic who testified to her faith and the connection with psychoanalysis in her book, *The Jesus of Psychoanalysis: A Freudian Interpretation of the Gospel*. Lacan himself repeatedly uses biblical motifs ranging from Abraham to St Paul, a figure also much vaunted by the Lacanian philosopher Alain Badiou, albeit as an atheist, and by Žižek, who, I suspect, will convert to Christianity on his deathbed.

Lacan's take on Freud's *Beyond the Pleasure Principle* is to point to a form of excessive enjoyment that shades into pain, *jouissance*, which he ruminates on at some length in his discussion of St Teresa; and this fuels the devout readings of Lacan as a kind of Christian sage who is showing us how 'castration' is the cut into illusory plenitude of the subject, a version of original sin and separation from God's love, from the Other. One might, then, see Lacan as indicative of a second-wave Christianising of psychoanalysis as it becomes at one with the culture it is supposed to refuse adaptation to. This adaptation and Christianising of psychoanalysis then run alongside the popular diffusion of Freudian motifs into mass culture, motifs that do not disturb that culture but confirm its power. As that happens, as psychoanalysis is turned into something that is the same as the dominant culture instead of being resistant to it, new forms of otherness appear. Otherness is displaced onto 'other' cultures.

Ummah

Between them Sabah Siddiqui and João Gabriel Lima da Silva provoked the thought that there may be a third wave of psychoanalysis in which Islam would play a key role, and that either the task was to look for forms of 'psychoanalytic Islam' or to develop forms of 'Islamic psychoanalysis' – or both. For João from Brazil, which was a context in which psychoanalysis has always been implicitly linked with religion, this would be a way, perhaps, of taking psychoanalysis forward. As in many other parts of the world, the first wave of psychoanalysis was facilitated in Brazil by Jewish émigrés from continental Europe. While these analysts were themselves usually secular Jews, the practice was viewed as something 'other'. The assimilation of psychoanalysis to the eclectic mixture of therapeutic approaches in Brazil was achieved when the second generation of psychoanalysts appeared, with the first leading figure of the Lacanian movement a Mother Superior. But now there might, perhaps, be something of the syncretism that Chris Dunker described in a third wave of psychoanalysis, one that was able to link with Islam.

Why not bring together psychoanalysts, psychoanalytic researchers and Islamic scholars and those working at the interface of these traditions of work together in a conference in Manchester? That would be one way of approaching the question. Instead of trying to fuse them together, we would need instead, in the spirit of Deleuze and Guattari's anti-Oedipal 'schizoanalysis', to construct assemblages in which they operated together.

Sabah Siddiqui was carrying out research at a Muslim shrine in Gujarat, a strongly Hindu nationalist state in India, political base of Narendra Modi, the current prime minister. She was up for a conference on the intersection between Islam and psychoanalysis not only because of the way that Islam was being demonised as 'other' to Hindu culture under Modi, but also because it was being made the prime target of the psychiatric medicalisation of distress. There were plenty of Hindu temples in India that were site of healing rituals to which people in distress went, alternative approaches drawing on religious practices that could complement medical psychiatry. For the activists in the so-called 'anti-superstition' movement, this complementary approach was itself, problematic, for they wanted such healing practices replaced with tested, scientific treatments. For the Hindu state, however, the most dangerous forms of superstition were to be found not in the Hindu temples, but in the Muslim shrines, and so particular attention was given to those sites. Psychiatric clinics would be set up near the shrines, in some cases inside them. Sabah Siddiqui's concern was not with romanticising the shrines, for some of their religious healing practices are quite violent, but with how psychoanalysis might play a non-medical role in relation to those healing practices. So, you see two quite different contexts – Brazil and India – in which this question of the relationship between Islam and psychoanalysis would play out.

In Britain, where we decided to hold the conference, there is yet another context, one of increasing suspicion bordering on hatred of Muslims that has in the last decade been increasingly conceptualised as 'Islamophobia'. The 'phobia' that is referred to here is as reductionist and psychologising as when it is made to signify homophobia, but it does capture something of the structural symbolic conditions in which Muslims often encounter non-Muslims in the West. Terrorist attacks in the United States, on mainland Europe and in Britain have increased the atmosphere of threat, threat experienced by Muslims targeted with new security measures and threat experienced by those confronted with signs of community enclosure that, they have been told by the mass media, amount to fanaticism. There have been suggestions that women should be made to go unveiled in public places in Britain in recent years, as there have been in France, and even suggestions in France among some secular psychoanalysts that the veil is an obstacle to communication, a particularly bizarre claim when made by those who use the couch as a mechanism to break the Imaginary in the clinic.

To hold such a conference at this time would also be a political act, and as such would be a clear public statement about where psychoanalysis stands, with the Muslim community rather than against them, declaring that they were allies instead of enemies. This raises a general question about where psychoanalysts stand on political matters, and where 'analytic neutrality' in the clinic is assumed to be something that must be transposed to the exterior symbolic space that makes it possible. On a personal level I am guessing that most if not all of my current analysands will know something about my politics. Most refer to it or hint at it. This observation calls for a short intermission in this chapter for a couple of pages, a diversion, so we can then return to think about some of the consequences of having a public conference on such a topic.

There had been some dramatic changes in the context for my clinical work in the previous few years. First with a shift from the speech pathology clinic to my own office in Manchester Metropolitan University, MMU, after the clinic became too noisy at times and I was worried about people intruding into the clinical space from the corridors; then a shift from one office to another, with my new bare room most unappealing, small, difficult to arrange the chairs so that it would be possible to position my analysands as if they were on a couch; and then the shift out of MMU when I was aware that there could, at any moment, be an attempt by management to close it down. In a pre-emptive move, I searched for a clinical space outside the university. I didn't want it in my own house because I wanted to keep home life separate from work, and whatever my analysands knew about my academic or political work, I had, at least, managed to keep my personal life shielded, more enigmatic we might say. Things came to a head in a public trade union dispute in which I was singled out by management as threat and example.

I contacted a private health clinic that included acupuncture, physiotherapy and cognitive behavioural treatments, but was told that the psychologists would find the presence of a psychoanalyst disturbing. Then I found a local hypnotherapy centre, which was in a large family house in a leafy side road. In fact, it was the large family house, and patients were led through the hallway, past the two cats, and into a sitting room with two large comfortable sofas facing each other. This was not perfect, but it would have to do. Meanwhile I applied to hire a room in a local psychoanalytic psychotherapy clinic. I had applied for space there as soon as I had completed my training back in 2004, but my application had been blocked, I was told by an inside source, by the IPA psychoanalyst John Churcher, who was still smarting from our conflict over representations of psychoanalytic training. Even before that, my response to a request to hire a room there five years earlier had been rebuffed because I was not yet registered and also because, as they put it in their letter replying to my request, 'practitioners already working here reserve the right to ensure that boundaries can be preserved whenever an application is made'. By now, late 2012, John Churcher had moved out of this clinic after some disagreements over the sanctity of the clinical room. Apparently, one day he had come in to find a large sooty footprint on the couch he used, a footprint made by a workman getting access to the loft.

My analysands obediently relocated from MMU to a hypnotherapy centre, intrigued by the name of the place when I told them the address, and they speculated much about whether this was my own house. I didn't confirm or deny it. We don't do that. Such questions are always the opportunity for the analyst to ask further questions, not to answer them, and questions always reveal something of the internal life of the analysand. Clinical structure as such is always haunted by a question, a question for the hysteric as to whether they are a man or a woman, and for the obsessional as to whether they are alive or dead. The pervert, if there is such a clinical structure, which I have now come to doubt, would want to know how to make the other exist and be an instrument of the deadly excessive enjoyment of the other – that which Lacan names '*jouissance*'. The psychotic, another clinical structure I am agnostic about, would not have a question, and that is a problem that indicates, to the psychoanalyst who believes in it, that such a structure is present.

Is such a structure really present? By now I was not so sure. The label 'psychotic' has often been a signifier in a deadly life sentence handed to patients by psychiatrists as well as, shame on them, by some psychoanalysts. It has also been a label used to exclude some people from psychoanalytic training. A psychotic analyst is unthinkable. I was much affected by the conceptual clinical transition to Lacan's work described by Annie Rogers in her marvellous 2006 book *The Unsayable: The Hidden Language of Trauma*, a book I would henceforth recommend to practising psychotherapists as an introduction to Lacanian work. The blurry misery-lit image on the front cover of the first edition of the book put me off reading it after Carol Owens gave me a copy during a visit to Dublin, a place Annie Rogers often visits to speak about her work, but Carol insisted I give it a go, and I am glad I did. When I did read it I was stunned by the clarity of the writing and depth of engagement with the language of 'psychosis'. Along the way in the narrative, Annie discloses that she herself acquired a diagnosis of psychosis, and, yes, she believes it, believes in the existence of that clinical structure, but she claims it and uses it in the clinic in such a way as to deconstruct, de-pathologise it. Her work with the Freudian School of Quebec deepened an approach to psychosis that breaks from the medical model. She shows us how, whether it really exists or not, the clinical coordinates that Lacanian notions of 'structure' provide can help the analyst, and help the analyst provide a supportive space for their analysands to speak. This is more helpful than recent assumptions made by some Lacanians, followers of Jacques-Alain Miller, that if there is no direct indication of neurotic or perverse structure then there must, by default, be psychotic structure, what they call 'ordinary psychosis.'

The phrasing of a question can indicate something of the structure, there being a marked difference between an analysand wanting to know if this is my family home, for example, hysteric perhaps, or wanting to know how I manage my life in the house, perhaps obsessional. If there are no such questions then that does indicate a problem, if you are to believe some psychoanalysts. I arrived at the hypnotherapy centre one day just before Christmas to be warned by the owner and lead hypnotherapist that I might find that there had been some changes in the sitting room. There were. The place was festooned with Christmas cards and a large plastic silver Christmas tree with decorations and lights dripping off it. My analysands raised their eyebrows, but the fact that they didn't say anything probably indicated how really weird this was.

By the time I did manage to get my room for rent approved in the local psychotherapy clinic, news of the trade union dispute I had been involved in at MMU had been made public, with articles in local and national newspapers. I moved some analysands to my new clinical space, but they didn't stay much longer, the analysis had been disrupted too much, and the new analysands that I took on were, in different ways, already cued into what had happened at MMU and why I had left it. In some cases, analysands referred to political reasons for beginning analysis, implicit identification either with my situation or directly with me in the preliminary sessions. Psychoanalytic organisations, including my training organisation, CFAR, and the LSNLS and the College of Psychoanalysts supported me, and I was able to carry on attending psychoanalytic meetings, a calming alternative base for my thinking and writing.

In addition to these institutional forms of solidarity were symbolic forms of support. The Symbolic provides the guide rails for life for us, for human subjects as social beings. My friend Antony Easthope learnt to drive late in life, and would describe his surprise at how important the system of traffic and car indicator signals were: "It really is a matter of life and death," he used to say, "it is just like the Symbolic, one false move and you're dead." The Laibach track 'The Whistle-blowers', on their album *Spectre*, became for me a retroactive emblem of what I had been through in what was to become properly 'traumatic'; at some early point, on hearing the track, I was overwhelmed with emotion, sucked back into the events, raising questions about how I succeeded or failed in following Laibach's strategy of 'over-identification' as a way of dealing with power. There it is a discursive repetition of what power wants you to do, but in such a way that it rubs what is wrong with that in their faces, in a manner very close to what used to be treated as an element of insubordination in the army and called 'dumb insolence'. The difference being that over-identification in which you mimic what you are expected to say, perform in line with the way you are expected to behave, is not a 'psychological' phenomenon. It is not inside the head as 'identification' with another you are closely and emotionally linked with, not private as it is usually assumed to be, but public, and even more so when you make visible the aspects of it that are usually kept hidden, when you are a whistleblower.

I also, soon after these dramatic life changes, and connected with them, took on a more prominent role in the College of Psychoanalysts, through which I had helped organise a conference at the LSE on psychoanalysis and state regulation with Simona Revelli in 2006, and then we edited a book of papers from the conference. The book was good, a useful intervention, but it was difficult to get people to publicly endorse it. Susie Orbach replied, 'not really my area', but 'good luck with it'. Peter Fonagy, head of research at the IPA, was unable to write something, his secretary said, 'due to the pressure of prior commitments'. Fonagy had already, rather scandalously, ditched the notion of the unconscious in order to make psychoanalysis palatable to neuroscientists, and he developed forms of psychotherapy compatible with the new regulatory bodies and the health service administrators. These new forms of therapy included 'Mentalization-based treatment', MBT, an approach he cooked up with Anthony Bateman. Patients would effectively be told how they could or should feel about key events in their lives or about their relationships with others.

This approach continued the worst of Donald Winnicott's lectures on BBC radio to young mothers from 1943 to 1962. At one event in Manchester, chaired by Steve Potter of the University Counselling Service, for example, Bateman cradled an imaginary baby in his arms and kissed and cooed at it to show us what real nurturing behaviour looked like – 'mansplaining' in action. The appeal to neuroscience is mostly bogus, and draws tendentious parallels between what we see and what is picked up in functional Magnetic Resonance Imaging brain scans; as Erica Burman pointed out in a paper in the journal *Group Analysis*, even scans of a dead salmon have been shown to show significant brain activity. We are subjects not brains, and it is as subjects that we speak to the psychoanalyst in the clinic. The reduction of us to our brains is of a piece with scientistic specification and regulation of what we are and what we could be. That reductive approach is, as Jan de Vos points out, 'neurologisation' that gives another bizarre twist to contemporary psychologisation of clinical and everyday experience. We had an honest response to our request for a blurb on the back cover of our book on state regulation from the novelist Hanif Kureishi, who wrote 'I found the writing so obscure, the prose so intransigent and the arguments so elliptical I couldn't possibly recommend it to anyone. If this is where psychoanalysis is today I can't see what meaning it could have for the general public.' Oh well, you can't win them all.

The book launch was at Freud's house in Maresfield Gardens. Simona Revelli arranged the Laurie Anderson sarcastic music video 'Only an Expert' to play on a loop, and we ranged around the house from the garden where the food and drink was to the green-and-white-tiled bathroom upstairs. An ebullient Brazilian visitor – you can guess who – dared to lie on the famous couch while friends and family took photos. At the end of the evening, as dusk fell and we gathered up the debris, we felt we were surrounded by ghosts, whether we liked it or not, whether we believed in them or not. These were our ghosts, the traces of the past and the networks of colleagues who made this strange practice, the talking cure, possible.

That was a time of strange alliances, including with Jungian Andrew Samuels, who had been given an honorary fellowship at one of the ghastly United Kingdom Council for Psychotherapy (UKCP) meetings at which I represented CFAR. In a 2009 email to treasure, Andrew wrote to me about squabbles in the Society for Analytical Psychology and the IPA's own registration front-organisation (now the BPC) and about his recent election as Chair of UKCP; 'This is all your fucking fault, Ian, because when I got my Hon Fell of UKCP in 2006 you convinced me to turn against state reg.' Andrew was actively involved in the Alliance for Counselling and Psychotherapy, which brought together psychoanalytic types with humanists like Denis Postle to resist state regulation of our practice.

The last thing I wanted to do after I left MMU was go through those state regulation debates again ten years on, but the College, which brought together psychoanalysts who had not been trained by the IPA, asked me to get involved in it again. Simona Revelli persuaded me. I agreed to replace Darian Leader as president when he stepped down in 2015. I wanted to get the College actively involved in political questions. The first step had been to get it to explicitly back the first national conference of the Free Psychotherapy Network, which we held in Manchester in 2016; and now the second step would be to get it to stump up some money for the conference 'Islamic Psychoanalysis / Psychoanalytic Islam' the following year. Now we were back on track, almost, for the conference, which is where this long and winding introduction to the main topic of this chapter has been leading.

We had a discussion about this at the 2016 Annual General Meeting, where Richard Klein, who had by now left the London Society to set up his own outfit called The School of the Freudian Letter, intervened with a typically cryptic comment designed to hystericise the audience: "You could invite the police," he said. I was chairing the meeting, and asked him why. "Well," he said, "the police would be very interested in such matters and would have a lot to learn." I was flustered, the group was anxious, Richard was amused. We got approval for funding for advertising, applied for more funding from the University of Manchester, which I was amazed to get agreement for, given the British government's 'hostile environment' for migrants strategy, and contacted likely participants.

We wanted to avoid inviting people or accepting papers that would simply give the stage for one side in the encounter to provide a metanarrative to explain to the other what they really meant; to avoid Islamic scholars lecturing us about why psychoanalysis was wrong; and to avoid psychoanalytic statements of the kind that had been made by Žižek, for example, that Islam is grounded on disavowed femininity. We took a risk inviting Fethi Benslama from Paris, suspecting that he would come at the question from the psychoanalytic metanarrative side of the argument, but in the event, after he accepted the invitation, he had to undergo a medical operation and Andrea Mura came in at a late stage to give a very good extemporised talk on the cultural discursive contexts for this encounter. Amal Treacher, an old ally from the days of the Free Associations conferences and then 'Flesh and Blood', now Amal Treacher Kabesh, gave the opening talk.

Gohar Homayounpour from Teheran was our third guest speaker. As a cosmopolitan subject who had trained as an IPA psychoanalyst in the US and flitted backwards and forwards across the Atlantic, she had no problem getting a visa, unlike every other speaker who submitted papers from Iran; they were refused entry to the UK. Nevertheless, we did have speakers from Brazil, Germany, Greece, India, Iran, Ireland, Italy, Mexico, Turkey, the US and, of course, the UK. Brazilian João could not be there, he was back in Rio waiting on the birth of his first child, and he had also changed his mind about the basis of the conference, now arguing that only psychoanalysis allows us to comprehend the nature of religious experience, whether that is Judaism, Christianity or Islam. Well, back on track with the main line with the mainstream psychoanalytic tradition then.

Gohar Homayounpour's keynote paper was also one of the most controversial. She argued that it was in the nature of Islam to be cryptic and unfathomable to those who were not of the faith, or even for those who were – because of the privilege given to the Arabic text. The recitation of the Quran in Arabic as the voice of God and as the basis of religious practice cuts the Muslim off from whatever host culture they live in, and the radical refusal of translation poses a problem for non-Muslims and Muslims alike. Translation here is impossible. It is as if we are faced here with Arabic as a 'wall of language' that shields the Muslim from the rest of the world. Sabah fumed.

I am not sure, first, whether this is very different from many other religious traditions that look back to founding texts, which they obsessively circle around. More than that, I am not sure that it differs so much from our day-to-day practices of reading about psychoanalysis. We were faced in this conference, and then in the book of the event, with a question about the non-relation between psychoanalysis and Islam as a faith that invites and then refuses to be deciphered. This was a question that led us to a deeper question about the nature of psychoanalysis itself as a faith that invites and refuses to be deciphered. Psychoanalysts who want to speak about the uncanny, for example, will routinely employ the original German term *Unheimlich* to capture something of the ambivalent contradictory meanings embedded in it, only able to evoke that by retreating to German. For Lacanians, this impossibility of translation is doubled, so that we add to *Nachträglichkeit* to evoke 'afterwardsness', *après-coup*, aftershock, and we have our own peculiar terms like *jouissance* and *objet petit a*. Is there not always a 'wall of language'?

The language of psychoanalysis is extremely useful, indispensable to make sense of the clinical practice that it conditions and frames, but it is surely a leap of faith to leap into that system of signifiers as the only vocabulary for making sense of subjectivity. Islam provides one overarching narrative for some believers, and for many psychoanalysts their own discourse is the one and only frame to make sense of life inside and outside the clinic. Are these the only frames? I don't believe it. Rather, we need to notice the limits of those frames if we are to better know what it is we are doing. This, at root, is an ethical question, a question about psychoanalytic practice in specific contexts that cannot be solved by an appeal to science or to state authorities that pretend to know what is good for us. A question I will use as the frame for the final chapter.

20

TRANSFERENCE

Ethics in action

Should members of the public be protected from psychoanalysts? Psychoanalysis is not a science – it is, Lacan says, 'a babbling practice' – so it is not clear what kind of criteria could ever be used to govern it, criteria that the psychoanalysts would accept. The truth that is spoken in the clinic is not verified empirically, but instead, Lacan says, has the 'structure of fiction', a poetic evocation of a subject who always escapes the regulative nature of language, and, more so, escapes the attempts by the state to turn ethics into a closed system of moral rules. It is not clear what we are to do about this irresolvable conflict between diametrically opposed agendas for treatment, whether we should bring people into line or create a space for them to speak. I warn you that, since this is my last chance in the book to tell you that we create spaces for people to speak, I rant a bit towards the end. What did you expect?

Ethics

I walk twenty minutes to the psychotherapy clinic early on a Friday morning. Past the synagogue on one side and past Kleinian John's house on the other, turn the corner, and past where Wittgenstein once lived when he studied aeronautical engineering in Manchester, and then past where Factory Records was founded. Hello to Eyal, taking son Joel to nursery on Burton Road, and then round to the left, into the driveway to unlock the door. I am the first one in today, open the blinds and turn on the light in the waiting room. Flick across the 'engaged' sign on the door of my room, Room 1, and put on the side-lights. I had a sharp-eyed analysand, David, who noticed that the main light was on one day, a bitter comment on things out of his control, that change without his knowing. His housemate also came for therapy here and loved the yellow William Morris print curtains. The dark magenta, cloth couch clashes with the faded pink carpet, covered with lines of intersecting grey dots, and there are some tacky pictures of Italian doors, and one of a cartoon cat, on the wall.

This is not really 'my' room, but one that has possessions of the psychiatrist member of the clinic collective on the shelves and leaflets giving advice about how to stop procrastinating in the desk drawers, a room that I live with; in fact I chose it because it is at ground level, close to the front door, even though the couch wall is next to the toilet, and analysands sometimes pause in their speech while listening to dribbling and splashing and flushing. All this kind of thing, this noise, is a reminder that the clinic is in the world, and, as we Lacanians often joke to each other, it is something to talk about.

This morning my first analysand, Mike, is a 'DNA', I picked that term up from my time at Gaskell House, and most therapists at this place who have worked in the NHS also know that it means 'Did Not Arrive', and so a cup of tea, arrival of some colleagues, and an annoyed insistent knocking on the door. When I open it, because the receptionist is not there yet, an elderly man is there with, I assume, his wife, complaining that the bell is not working "and it was not working last week," he says as he glares at me. A colleague, his therapist I guess, appears beside me to welcome them in. "Oh," she says to the woman, "You must be Jill, I'm so glad you were able to come here this week," so maybe this is some kind of couple therapy, and the therapist is being super nice; I suspect she is going to have a hard time. My second analysand arrives, Dawn, a chatty woman who has complained for four years that she has nothing to say, and that her friends – she has no friends she says – know it. She settles onto the couch and tells me that at the end of the last session she noticed that I looked annoyed and that she suspects I want to get rid of her.

I tell my analysands in the first session we meet that I will end our meetings at some time around thirty minutes, or a little less, or perhaps even a little more, and that ending the session in this way enables me to mark something important in what they are saying without spelling things out, and I tell them that the analysis ends when they leave, not when I tell them that their problem is cured. That decision to end it is up to them, a responsibility that they have to take, to decide and to tell me. My third analysand that morning, Peter, is a therapist, sensitive to being ignored, and tells me of a flash of rage he experienced when I collected him from the waiting room instead of meeting him at the front door, which I usually do, because he is usually dead on time. He tells me, after he has lain down, that he feels unsettled because his own supervisor had said to him about one of his difficult patients "Just take the money and let them talk." Peter does not need to spell out what he is thinking about. There is a silence, and I say "go on," and he laughs.

Some of my analysands speak about Freud and some of them speak about Lacan, and some of them just want to talk. Some of them are very aware of when I smile and when I frown, or when they imagine that I am doing so, and some of them tell me what they think about that. Some of them don't like the chatty therapeutic interaction they witness as my colleagues collect their patients from the waiting room, and some of them have told me outright at the beginning of the analysis that they are glad I am a Lacanian because that means that there is no chance of us two having a relationship. A sense of containment and security in the clinic clearly means different things to different people, and I have to be clear that I can guarantee nothing. I can listen. The ethics that suffuse our practice do not form a system of rules, and if they did I suspect that they would no longer be ethical. They would, perhaps, then function as a series of moral codes, even of regulations designed to make people behave well, but then analysts and analysands would just behave according to the rules, moral but not ethical.

The College of Psychoanalysts recently responded to the latest attempt to regulate our practice. I wrote the response after procrastinating, sick at returning to this debate after the last round of battles a decade ago during which we held the College 'Psychoanalysis and State Regulation' conference. That was a conference that ended with squabbles between two French analysts from different organisations, one accusing the other of collaborating with the state by agreeing to sign up to some new proposed regulatory frameworks. I chaired a small College open board meeting where some familiar faces appeared, older and deafer, Richard Klein the Lacanian and Bob Young the Kleinian – Bob having burnt his boats with the IPA after writing a paper about them, delightfully subtitled 'The Grand Leading the Bland' – the two analysts from quite different traditions of work speaking at cross purposes at the open meeting, wilfully misunderstanding each other, steadfastly staying on one combative version of the line of the Imaginary.

One subtext of the regulation of psychotherapy in the UK is usually an attempt by the IPA to shut out the Lacanians, or anyone who has not trained at the Institute of Psychoanalysis, and so it is important that the Bobs and the Richards should work together. The fantasy of regulation is that it will prevent people from doing bad things, even though there is already legal recourse to prosecute people who have engaged in financial or sexual exploitation or physical abuse. Worse than that, this fantasy that state regulation will save us fuels the illusion that those who are on an official 'register' of some kind will be a safe bet, that a patient will be safe in their hands. The last stab at regulation, which was by a Conservative government, conjured up the case of the family doctor Harold Shipman in north Manchester who murdered elderly patients, but failed to note that Shipman was actually registered with the General Medical Council.

Regulation would serve to specify who is a psychoanalyst, who is a therapist and who is a counsellor. One of the registration bodies keen to get the ear of government tried to sort out who is who with the very neat suggestion that counsellors see clients once a week, psychodynamic counsellors see them twice a week, psychotherapists see patients three times a week, psychoanalytic psychotherapists see them four times a week, and psychoanalysts see their analysands five times a week. I kid you not. In the last round of the battle over state regulation, psychotherapy was treated as a 'health profession', and at one point it was seriously proposed that practitioners should have a washing basin in their room and hang their certificate on the wall. This pigeon-holing of all psychotherapeutic work as a health profession was successfully resisted by the Alliance for Counselling and Psychotherapy and by the judicial review in 2011 demanded by the College of Psychoanalysts – UK. I doubted that it would work, and I was unsure that we should put our energies into a legal challenge, but in fact it worked out well, it was the right thing to do.

The Alliance was able, during that campaign, to transcend divisions between counsellors (of whom about 44,000 are registered with the British Association for Counselling and Psychotherapy), psychotherapists (8,000 are with the United Kingdom Council for Psychotherapy) and psychoanalysts (some of whom like to cling to their status, treating their small number, counted in the hundreds in Britain, as further evidence of eminence). The British Psychoanalytic Council goes so far as to prohibit dual membership with a rival body, mixing with the lower classes. Some budding bureaucrats in the registration bodies – the BACP, UKCP and the BPC – would like to tell you what you are and define what you get up to in the consulting room. These bodies already specify who is entitled to act as a supervisor for your work, and how you should keep notes from your sessions. We are expected to report analysands who say things that indicate that they might harm others, or harm themselves, to the authorities, and we may be required to hand over our notes. No dreams here please. A friend posted on Facebook about one of their encounters in the clinic with a cognitive behavioural therapist: "Therapist: have you ever thought about harming anyone else? Me, socialist intellectual: of course."

I was very impressed by IPA psychoanalyst André Green at a meeting about supervision in London. He spent the first part of the meeting complaining that Bernard Burgoyne, who was chairing the meeting, called himself a psychoanalyst, and reminded the audience that although he, André Green, had attended Lacan's seminars he was not a Lacanian. The IPA analysts were delighted, until Green lambasted attachment theory – "It's not attachment, it's love" – and then turned his attention to Donald Winnicott, pointing out that Winnicott had not been able to consummate his marriage until after his father died. What kind of psychoanalyst is that? Well, probably one somewhere within the normal range of odd people who train to do this kind of thing. A supervisee turned up to see Green with a handful of notes about the patient they wanted to talk about. "Put them away," Green said. "Your patient is not there," he said, pointed to the notes, "they should be *here*," he said as he banged his chest. That was that. He was right. Now I don't keep notes, but instead I have scattered jottings of key signifiers to anchor discussion of ongoing cases in my supervision sessions, jottings that would be meaningless to a third party and that are dispensed with as soon as they have served their purpose.

Of course there is abuse in psychotherapy, and this abuse has much to do with the nature of transference and how it is handled inside and outside the clinic. I suspect that the 'subject supposed to know' who appears inside the clinic is a function of the quite peculiar explicit and implicit rules of speech we follow there, but that 'transference' as such does not really exist outside it. There are some unscrupulous therapists who do their best in contained cult-like settings to evoke transference, but the issue there is really to do with power and the abuse of power, power we can better understand in terms of patriarchy and racism, and the systematic disempowerment of people who are positioned as vulnerable and expected to behave like victims.

There is a lesson here from the Hearing Voices movement. They point out that many people hear voices, sometimes experienced as friends or guides, and that the voices themselves are not necessarily the problem. Neighbours sometimes say nasty and upsetting things, but this does not mean that no one should have a neighbour. Similarly, the kinds of power to which we are subject, as well as what we call 'transference' inside the clinic, are forms of relationships we must learn to negotiate, rather than attempt to wish them away, as regulation of psychotherapy often tries to do. The question is how we account for what we experience, and how those who listen are made accountable.

Privacy

What is peculiar about the psychoanalytic clinic is precisely that it is an enclosed private space. The conditions of possibility for such a space, shut off from the collective shared to-and-fro of human interaction, are precisely the conditions of possibility for much distress under contemporary capitalism; alienation and isolation of people from each other. Wilhelm Reich tried to open this space up in the Sex-Pol movement, collectivising distress and mobilising those who had turned in on themselves, addressing his polemics against fascism to the 'little man' who replaced his failure with overweening fantasies of power over others and identification with leaders who would compensate for his castration and provide a vicarious sense of achievement. Erich Fromm complements this explicitly political mobilisation of human beings as collective subjects with appeals to the sense we have that our being is depleted the more we have; he argues that this is a false solution, and that spiritual enlightenment must proceed by way of a deeper relatedness of people to each other and to nature. For Fromm, psychoanalysis is one of the names for that spiritual path that people are searching for.

The ethical commitment of psychoanalysts to listen to those who want a space to speak in confidence about themselves, what Lacan calls the 'desire of the analyst', a desire to open a space for people to speak and to hear themselves say things they have never said before and to hear the connections between signifiers that they have never noticed before, is tied up with 'accountability'; this is accountability in the sense of being accountable and also in the sense of being able to give account of who one is. Again, the boundaries between the inside and the outside of the clinic, artificial boundaries that make of psychoanalysis a problem as well as a resource, are handled differently by different analysts.

I have heard psychoanalysts say that their patients were well or badly dressed or that young men were fat or thin, women pretty or ugly, and so on. I heard Donald Meltzer, a prominent 'post-Kleinian' psychoanalyst speak about clinical cases at a day conference organised by the North West Regional Psychotherapy Association, held at Gaskell House in May 1996. He was committed to psychoanalysis as a world view, and argued quite explicitly, when I asked him, that child development as described by Melanie Klein was universal; he had travelled the world and had seen no instances where it did not apply. An early episode of the original *Star Trek*,

'Metamorphosis', had a scientist character declare that gender is a universal construct applicable to all alien life forms as well as human beings. Some of the statements by psychoanalysts on this world are still light years out of date, and more insulting. Meltzer sat on the little stage and spoke as he unrolled and re-rolled a cigarette with his eyes closed, telling us that he had chosen three patients to talk about, "none of whom," he said, "are nice people." One of his cases was a young man who was a pervert who walked mud into the consulting room, made the carpet dirty and did not seem to care about that, Meltzer said. Meltzer told us that there was a fine painting hanging over his couch, a beautiful countryside scene, and that this young man had never, in all the years of analysis, commented on the painting. "The next patient I will tell you about," Meltzer said before the break, "is a real shocker with a gold ring through his nose and long hair, an Oxford student who spoke like a yob."

I have had some real characters speak to me in my clinic, but that is what people are supposed to be, characters. This is their chance to go beyond who they usually are, one of the joys of psychoanalysis. I have been shouted at in the clinic, and Dave, an actor, gave a very realistic performance of someone suffering post-traumatic flashbacks to being stabbed. I think he was annoyed when I didn't flinch, and more annoyed, he said, that I didn't laugh. Psychoanalysis is underwritten by a kind of pact that both the analysand and the analyst will speak very differently inside the clinic, and this sometimes has what psychiatrists called 'decompensating' effects outside it.

I was on a CFAR panel chaired by Darian Leader and Anouchka Grose in March 2018, with the writer Will Self, someone whose name consists of two potent signifiers, and he knows this. I busily prepared my paper for the panel, delighted that Self would be there to listen to it and say nice things about it. Some psychoanalysts would say that this was transference. In the event, it turned out that he was going to speak first and then leave early. Will Self read out a short article he had written and had already published about Donald Trump and sewers and shit before Trump's election. Self's microphone hovered over the stand briefly when he finished before he pulled it back to berate the audience for not laughing: "You miserable lot," he said, "it's what I would expect of you psychoanalysts." He continued in a long tirade against us all.

"I bet you don't talk about yourselves in the consulting room," he said, and I agreed. "Well," he said, "I want an analyst who will talk about their sex lives if I am going to talk about mine." That's fine, I pointed out, but then you would have a shared understanding or rivalrous banter on what we call the line of the Imaginary, maybe that's what you want, but it wouldn't be psychoanalysis. Will Self is tall. He towered above me. I felt rather frightened. "I know about psychoanalysis," Self said, "I was practically born in the toilets of the Tavistock Clinic." He then told us a remarkable story, which I'll bet he had rehearsed many times before, of how he had a copy of a letter that his mother's analyst, Anthony Storr, had sent her in which Storr had congratulated Self's mother for following his advice not to have an abortion. What is remarkable about this is not only the story as such, but the context in which Self was happy to tell it. Anthony Storr, well there's a thing, many people, and not only psychoanalysts would have heard of him. Some psychoanalysts would call it transference. Self then told us he had to leave for another meeting, and told us that he loved us all.

The kind of private space that psychoanalysts often defend is exactly the privatised space of the clinic as something sacrosanct, which is then replicated in clinical case presentation meetings. Darian once stopped a session in CFAR when he realised that someone was recording it, demanded the cassette tape be handed over, and exclaimed, "This is a clinical case!" Quite right. We are expected to change significant details in order to protect the confidentiality of the case, but too often we confuse confidentiality with anonymity. We think that by anonymising a case, concealing identifying marks from it, we are also being more confidential, when anonymity usually provides licence for more gossip and speculation – gossip and speculation, which is the most interesting talk in and around many psychoanalytic meetings.

One of the ways through this, taking a different path that reconfigures what psychoanalysis is as a social and political practice, has been explored by the Free Psychotherapy Network, FPN, which had its first national conference in Manchester in 2016. The conference was called 'Mind the Gap: Free Psychotherapy in an Unjust World'. The ethos of FPN picks up from humanistic and socialist psychotherapy traditions, and also from the 'Free Clinics' that flourished in Vienna, Berlin and Budapest in the 1920s and 1930s. One of the fetishes of contemporary psychoanalysis is that payment by the analysand is necessary for the particular kind of contract between analysand and analyst to be formed that is the precondition for the transference. A study of NHS public service psychoanalytic practitioners and private practitioners found, not surprisingly, that those in private practice believed more strongly in the idea that payment was necessary, therapeutically necessary, they claimed. It is a founding principle of psychoanalysis, many analysts believe, that the analysand must pay, but this is simply untrue. Chris Dunker once told me that when he sees children in his clinic in São Paulo he asks them to give him something, which might even be a bus ticket. He knows transference is not about the money, but about the symbolic bond between analyst and analysand.

In her 2005 book *Freud's Free Clinics: Psychoanalysis and Social Justice, 1918–1938*, Elizabeth Danto shows how the free clinics movement went way beyond Wilhelm Reich's Sex-Pol interventions. She notes how Freud argued, in a speech to the Fifth International Psychoanalytical Association congress in Budapest in 1918, that the conditions were being put in place for a free public health service in Hungary that should, he said, also include free public provision of psychoanalytic treatment. By a curious twist of fate, bureaucratic management and introduction of charges for treatment were introduced by the Nazis when they seized power and took over the clinics in Berlin.

The Free Psychotherapy Network conference included discussion of the kind of restricted fake 'accountability' that private practice requires and incites, and it opened the way for thinking in a different way about the relationship between free association and free speech and about free open relationships in which psychoanalysis as such would no longer be needed. The conference included activists from the 'democratic psychiatry' movement, people who had been in the psychiatric system and survived it, and wanted something better than physical treatments. Freud also argued that psychoanalysis is one of the three 'impossible professions', alongside educating and governing. Perhaps, as Žižek once pointed out, repeating a dictum from Wilhelm Reich, psychoanalysis is impossible in the kind of society where it is necessary and only possible in the kind of society where it is unnecessary. In the meantime, until it is unnecessary, we have a practice of speaking that, despite the shenanigans of the psychoanalysts, is not only necessary but sometimes joyful. There may be no such thing as 'free association', but there is a peculiar addictive freedom in the attempt to follow that fundamental technical rule in the clinic and to discover something about yourself that no one else need ever know. Your analyst will show a weird interest in your dreams that encourages you to speak, something in stark contrast to friends and relatives who will be as quickly bored by them as they are by repeated viewings of your holiday photos.

I chose to go into psychoanalytic practice to find out about it from the inside, so I am immersed in this discourse a lot of the time, and psychoanalytic discourse pervades the media and everyday conversation. It was worth it, it is the stuff of life, the life that bubbles away in our speech even when the words we are forced to repeat are deadened by institutions concerned more with the reproduction of power and status than the creativity they claim to value in their mission statements. We are subjects, not of this rationalised, conscious stream of empty speech, but of the unconscious. The full speech of psychoanalysis rebels against what we have been told, against who we have been told we are. It cannot be completely wiped away. Even if people hate psychoanalysis, they still rail against it, and defend themselves against the kinds of ad hominem accusations that they imagine psychoanalysts would make against them for refusing to take it seriously. Psychoanalysis reflects the alienated conditions of life under capitalism and I suspect that it is also one of the conditions for us being able to speak and reflect on what it is to be a subject today, whether we like it or not.

Subjectivity

Psychoanalysis defines what subjectivity today looks like, and it is objection to the way that description slides into prescription that leads some writers, followers of Gilles Deleuze for example, to be suspicious of it, that also leads to some resistance, some hostility to psychoanalysis as such. But, again, this kind of objection rather misses the point. The issue is not whether you are against psychoanalytic ideas about subjectivity but, because they are inescapable, how you address them, how you address what their effects are. There are undoubtedly some positive effects, as many Deleuzians would also acknowledge, particularly in the Lacanian tradition, as well as in some other traditions of psychoanalytic work. I wonder what this account would look like if I had gone down the group analytic path instead of the Lacanian one – perhaps much the same. We have tried to maintain the dialogue between these two and other analytic currents in Manchester Psychoanalytic Matrix, MPM, a collection of cartels and seminars where we discuss theory and practice. The group analysis Friday seminars are currently hosted at Manchester University after Erica Burman relocated here.

MPM hosted a book launch in Manchester, in April 2018, for a book edited by the Dublin-based psychoanalysts Carol Owens and Stephanie Farrelly Quinn called *Lacanian Psychoanalysis with Babies, Children and Adolescents*. Carol Owens, who listens to people as they lie on the couch, now listens to me in supervision. One of the most striking things that shine through in that book is the difference between psychiatric and psychological notions of development and images of childhood on the one hand, and Lacanian psychoanalytic concerns with the nature, rights and responsibilities of the human subject on the other. Psychiatry and psychological notions are well- meaning but conditional, defining what a child's ability to choose might be at different ages, and stipulating certain kinds of treatment, and, of course, certain requisite 'competencies' of the therapist.

Against such moral regulatory and restricted humanist models of the child, the Lacanian psychoanalyst is actually much closer to the most humanist imaginable ethic, closer to a quasi-existentialist approach to each human subject in its singularity. I remember a French Lacanian at CFAR discussing her work in a hospital where a patient was wheeled in on a bed sedated, near to death, the bedclothes falling off her naked body. The nurses talked over her and treated her as an object, and the Lacanian shouted as she covered up the body "Listen to her, she is a *subject!*" The human being is a subject in the most profound philosophical sense of the term, a philosophical sense inherited from the Western Enlightenment tradition that made psychoanalysis possible.

This psychoanalytic sense of subjectivity is extended by writers like Slavoj Žižek, and, even more so, his brother in arms in their 'gang of two', Alain Badiou. Badiou draws attention to something implicit in Lacan's diagrams, including the Schema L and the four discourses, which is that subjectivity here is distributed not only over the 'matheme' elements but also over the social field. The terms are not confined inside the head of the individual subject, but map a space for subjectivity that is also exterior to the subject. To be 'subject' is not to be an individual, separate and undivided at all; psychoanalytically-speaking, the 'subject' is also something collective, and that understanding of what it is to be a subject opens up a completely different terrain of debate about what it is to be accountable, to be accountable to others and to give account of oneself.

This account of subjectivity can also even be found in the work of Lacanian psychoanalysts in an international network, the 'École lacanienne de psychoanalyse', which was founded in 1985 by Jean Allouch and his followers. Yes, this is yet another 'international' alongside those controlled by Jacques-Alain Miller, Colette Soler and Charles Melman. The so-called 'Allouchians' in this fourth international take an innovative tack on the definitions of clinical structure, clinical case presentation and the historical constitution of subjectivity. The triplet of clinical structures in much Lacanian practice, of neurosis, psychosis and perversion, are problematically normative, Allouch argues, and form a prescriptive complex that he calls the 'Pernepsy' complex – a contraction of the diagnostic triad Perversion

Neurosis Psychosis – something that he associates with the 'psy complex' that one finds analysed by followers of Michel Foucault.

Clinical case presentations organised around these clinical structures also mislead trainee analysts about the nature of the practice, its indeterminacy, unpredictability and its attention to the singularity of the subject. We learn from Foucault, and also from Judith Butler, Jean Allouch argues, that psychoanalysis has to be situated in a much broader political project, one that takes questions of discipline, confession and queer critique seriously. Maybe this book is Allouchian, maybe not enough or too much so. David Pavón Cuéllar tells me that many of his students in Morelia, Mexico, consider themselves to be Allouchians, but that even their essays can sometimes be conformist and dogmatic. So it goes.

I still go to meetings organised by CFAR, which steadfastly stands aside from these different internationals, and to meetings organised by Solerians and Millerians. I loved the Millerian announcement at the head of their online newsletter, *The Symptom*, based in the United States after Miller promised to conquer the English-speaking world: 'Universalism versus globalization. This will be our US chapter – to be read as United Symptoms'. This is very Laibachian. And I am intrigued by their turn to politics and the formation of ZADIG; the name is borrowed from a little novel by Voltaire, and is an acronym for Zero Abjection Democratic International Group. The Laboratory for Lacanian Politics, a new NLS front organisation run by Janet Low, now Haney, together with the NLS online publication, *Lacanian Review*, run some interesting pieces but still tend to reduce political phenomena to psychoanalytic symbolic coordinates. There was no reply, however, to the USA-Palestine Mental Health Network appeal I forwarded to the NLS, requesting that they move the site of their 2019 congress from Tel Aviv. There have been interesting developments as part of the recent 'turn to politics' by the Millerians, with the appearance of the Lacanemancipa project linked to the Argentinian analyst Jorge Alemán, a project that has as the subtitle of its bilingual English-Spanish magazine 'Against the one of capitalism, the not-all of emancipation'.

I am a divided subject. I divide my time between work in the clinic, research on the construction of subjectivity and political intervention, and this divided attention affects how I listen to my analysands, and how I listen to people who listen to analysands speak about what they do outside the clinic. We are all located in a range of different contradictory social practices that define subjectivity, practices that include transference but also go beyond it. We cannot pin down 'transference' as such, isolate it as if it occurs only inside the analysand, as they construct their own particular 'subject supposed to know' and orient themselves to something enigmatic in the analyst that we define as semblant of *objet petit a*. Transference isn't what people in the clinic think, it is something else entirely.

I walk home from the clinic on Friday afternoon. Shouting man is at the bus stop again. He shouts out, as if he wants someone to listen to him, but he is closed in on himself, closed in without access to the private clinic resources, and quite probably knowing very little about the work that goes on there. He lives in temporary accommodation on Palatine Road. The task here surely goes well beyond simply educating him to know how to ask for treatment, to make a 'demand' for psychoanalysis. It includes, as a necessary condition for that, dramatic cultural and political changes in the way we organise services and space for people to speak about themselves. The Lacanian psychoanalyst Octave Mannoni, someone that Frantz Fanon clashed with precisely because he was worth arguing with, wrote in his 1950 classic text *Prospero and Caliban* that the only genuinely collective psychotherapy is what is known as politics. The connection of psychoanalysis with politics has also been necessary in the solidarity events the College of Psychoanalysts has arranged with colleagues in Brazil under threat from the state following the election of Jair Bolsonaro.

Some would say that the question posed at the beginning of this chapter, as to whether the public should be protected from psychoanalysts should be rephrased so that we ask how the public should be protected from rogue psychoanalysts, or those that are unethical, or those that do not follow moral guidelines set in place by the appropriate regulatory bodies. The problem is not the rogue psychoanalysts, however but a problem that lies in wait for every psychoanalyst, tempting them to think they know more than they possibly can do about transference and the unconscious and the depths of the soul.

Institutional rules will not protect us against anxiety about bad things, abuse or death, we should have learned that much. Instead we need to listen to the different ethical positions enunciated by different subjects. Many of the figures you have met in this book are no longer with us. I will mention three. Antony Easthope died of a cancer that he said was inside him "like in the film *Alien*," he said, "it is going to get me but I'm not going without a fight." Sheila Ernst, the group analyst, convened a special group at the IGA where they discussed with her a decision she had already made to end her own life before succumbing to motor neurone disease. Joel Kovel went soon after completing his poignant autobiography, *The Lost Traveller's Dream*, a settling of accounts with psychoanalysis and politics and religion, becoming an Episcopalian toward the end of his life. "Maybe he was looking for dad," an IPA-analyst friend rather unkindly commented. I was writing a first draft of this book when I heard the news of Joel's death.

How dare they, those who turn psychoanalysis back into a form of psychiatric normative practice. How dare they tell us how we should live and what we should think. I have just watched again the BBC Television Lifeline programme called 'Mars and Venus Speak to Earth', broadcast in 1959, where David Stafford-Clark interviews Dr George King of the Aetherius Society. Another psychiatrist, Anthony Storr, is brought in towards the end of the programme to deliver his verdict in front of King, who is reduced to being a silent object, a dignified mad patient, who, Storr says, in his British upper-class cut-glass accent, is engaging in 'projection'. Stafford-Clark solemnly concurs as he closes the programme. No, I don't believe this London taxi driver and yoga adept was really in contact with aliens, but why should I even have to tell you that. My attachment to psychoanalysis is not to it as a science but as a powerful fiction; why not declare that Lacan's take on Freud is a form of science fiction, and no less radical and transformative for that. Another world is possible, many worlds.

Psychoanalysis sets itself against those apparatuses, ideologies and powerful individuals who say that they know how we think. They do not know how people think, and neither should you think you can know how people think, by learning about psychoanalysis, by learning how to 'psychoanalyse' other people. Psychoanalysis is not what you think; it challenges, subverts the very idea, challenges and subverts each and every normative notion about subjectivity. That is what makes it radical, and that is why I remain committed to it as one among many different radical frameworks for grasping what it is to be a human being.

BIBLIOGRAPHY

Adorno, T. W. and Horkheimer, M. (1944/1979) *Dialectic of Enlightenment*. London: Verso.

Akeret, R. (1997) *The Man Who Loved a Polar Bear: And Other Psychotherapist's Tales* (new edition). Harmondsworth, UK: Penguin.

Allouch, J. (2014) 'Fragilities of analysis', *The Letter: Lacanian Perspectives on Psychoanalysis*, 57, pp. 29–40.

Althusser, L. (1971) *Lenin and Philosophy, and Other Essays*. London: New Left Books.

Bakan, D. (1958/1990) *Sigmund Freud and the Jewish Mystical Tradition*. London: Free Association Books.

Barnes, B., Ernst, S. and Hyde, K. (1999) *An Introduction to Groupwork: A Group-Analytic Perspective*. Basingstoke, UK: Palgrave.

de Beauvoir, S. (1949/1968) *The Second Sex*. London: Jonathan Cape.

Berne, E. (1964) *Games People Play: The Psychology of Human Relationships*. New York: Grove Press.

Bettelheim, B. (1986) *Freud and Man's Soul*. Harmondsworth: Pelican.

Bion, W. and Rickman, J. (1943) 'Intra-group tensions in therapy', *Lancet*, 2, pp. 678–681.

Burman, E. (2011) 'Environ-mentalizing the matrix', *Group Analysis*, 44 (4), pp. 374–384.

Burman, E. (2019) *Fanon, Education, Action: Child as Method*. London and New York: Routledge.

Butler, J. (1990) *Gender Trouble: Feminism and the Subversion of Identity*. London and New York: Routledge.

Butler, J. (1993) *Bodies That Matter: On the Discursive Limits of 'Sex'*. London and New York: Routledge.

Butler, J., Laclau, E. and Žižek, S. (2000) *Contingency, Hegemony, Universality: Contemporary Dialogues on the Left*. London: Verso.

Cardinal, M. (2013) *The Words to Say It* (9th edition). Cambridge, MA: Van Vactor & Goodheart.

Craib, I. (1994) *The Importance of Disappointment*. London and New York: Routledge.

Danto, E. A. (2005) *Freud's Free Clinics: Psychoanalysis and Social Justice, 1918–1938*. New York: Columbia University Press.

De Vos, J. (2012) *Psychologisation in Times of Globalisation*. London and New York: Routledge.

De Vos, J. (2016) *The Metamorphoses of the Brain: Neurologisation and its Discontents*. London: Palgrave Macmillan.

Deleuze, G. and Guattari, F. (1972/1977) *Anti-Oedipus: Capitalism and Schizophrenia*. New York: Viking.

Doi, T. (1971/1973) *The Anatomy of Dependence*. Tokyo: Kodansha International.

Dolto, F. (1979) *The Jesus of Psychoanalysis: Freudian Interpretation of the Gospel*. New York: Doubleday.

Dunker, C. (2010) *The Structure and Constitution of the Psychoanalytic Clinic: Negativity and Conflict in Contemporary Practice*. London: Karnac.

Elias, N. (1994) *The Civilizing Process*. Oxford: Blackwell.

Ernst, S. and Goodison, L. (1981) *In Our Own Hands: A Book of Self-Help Therapy*. London: The Women's Press.

Ernst, S. and Maguire, M. (eds) (1987) *Living with the Sphinx: Papers from the Women's Therapy Centre*. London: Women's Press.

Fanon, F. (1952/1967) *Black Skin, White Masks*. New York: Grove Press.

Forrester, J. (1980) *Language and the Origins of Psychoanalysis*. London: Macmillan.

Foucault, M. (1961/2009) *History of Madness*. London and New York: Routledge.

Foucault, M. (1975/1979) *Discipline and Punish: The Birth of the Prison*. Harmondsworth, UK: Penguin.

Foucault, M. (1976/1981) *The History of Sexuality, Vol. I: An Introduction*. Harmondsworth, UK: Pelican.

Foucault, M. (1984/1986) *The Care of the Self: The History of Sexuality, Vol. III*. Harmondsworth, UK: Penguin.

Foulkes, S. H. (1984) *Therapeutic Group Analysis*. London: Karnac.

Freud, A. (1936) *The Ego and the Mechanisms of Defence*. London: The Hogarth Press.

Freud, S. (1966–1974) *The Standard Edition of the Complete Psychological Works of Sigmund Freud* (translated by J. Strachey). London: Vintage, The Hogarth Press and the Institute of Psychoanalysis, 24 Vols.

Fromm, E. (1960) *Psychoanalysis and Zen Buddhism*. London: Unwin.

Fromm, E. (1974) *The Anatomy of Human Destructiveness*. London: Cape.

Frosh, S. (2002) *After Words: The Personal in Gender, Culture and Psychotherapy*. Houndmills, UK and New York: Palgrave Macmillan.

Fuller, P. (1980) *Art and Psychoanalysis*. London: Writers and Readers.

Gellner, E. (1985) *The Psychoanalytic Movement, or The Cunning of Unreason*. London: Paladin.

Giffney, N. and E. Watson, E. (eds) (2017) *Clinical Encounters in Sexuality: Psychoanalytic Practice and Queer Theory*. Goleta, CA: Punctum Books.

Gilman, S. (1991) *The Jew's Body*. London and New York: Routledge.

Henriques, J., Hollway, W., Urwin, C., Venn, C. and Walkerdine, V. (1984/1998) *Changing the Subject: Psychology, Social Regulation and Subjectivity*. London and New York: Routledge.

Hobson, R. F. (1985) *Forms of Feeling: The Heart of Psychotherapy*. London: Routledge.

Homayounpour, G. (2012). *Doing Psychoanalysis in Tehran*. Cambridge, MA: MIT Press.

Jacoby, R. (1983) *The Repression of Psychoanalysis*. New York: Basic Books.

Jaques, E. (1951) *The Changing Culture of a Factory*. London and New York: Routledge and Kegan Paul.

Kernberg, O. (1996) 'Thirty methods to destroy the creativity of psychoanalytic candidates', *International Journal of Psychoanalysis*, 77, pp. 1031–1040.

Klein, M. (1962) *Envy and Gratitude and Other Works, 1946–1963* (2nd edition). New York: Free Press.

Klein, M. (1932/1977) *The Psycho-Analysis of Children* (3rd edition). London: Vintage.

Kovel, J. (1978) *A Complete Guide to Therapy: From Psychoanalysis to Behaviour Modification*. Harmondsworth: Penguin.

Kovel, J. (1981) *The Age of Desire: Case Histories of a Radical Psychoanalyst.* New York: Pantheon.

Kovel, J. (1983) *Against the State of Nuclear Terror.* London: Pan.

Kovel, J. (1988) *White Racism: A Psychohistory.* London: Free Association Books.

Kovel, J. (2017) *The Lost Traveller's Dream: A Memoir.* Brooklyn, NY: Autonomedia.

Lacan, J. (1975/1998) *On Feminine Sexuality, The Limits of Love and Knowledge, 1972–1973: Encore, The Seminar of Jacques Lacan, Book XX.* New York: Norton.

Lacan, J. (1975–1976) *The Seminar of Jacques Lacan, Book XXIII: The Sinthome*, translated by C. Gallagher from unedited French manuscripts, at http://www.lacaninireland.com/web/translations/seminars/ (accessed 29 January 2019).

Lacan, J. (1991/2007) *The Other Side of Psychoanalysis: The Seminar of Jacques Lacan, Book XVII.* New York: W. W. Norton and Co.

Lacan, J. (1995) 'Proposition of 9 October 1967 on the psychoanalyst of the school', *Analysis*, 6, pp. 1–13.

Lacan, J. (2006) *Écrits: The First Complete Edition in English.* New York: Norton.

Laclau, E. and Mouffe, C. (1985). *Hegemony and Socialist Strategy: Towards a Radical Democratic Politics*, London: Verso.

Laplanche, J. (1989) *New Foundations for Psychoanalysis.* Oxford: Blackwell.

Laplanche, J. and Pontalis, J. B. (1988) *The Language of Psychoanalysis.* London: Karnac Books and the Institute of Psychoanalysis.

Lasch, C. (1978) *The Culture of Narcissism: American Life in an Age of Diminishing Expectations.* New York: Norton.

Lévi-Strauss, C. (1958/1972) *Structural Anthropology.* Harmondsworth, UK: Penguin.

Lindner, R. (1955/1986) *The Fifty-Minute Hour: A Collection of True Psychoanalytic Tales.* London: Free Association Books.

Macey, D. (1988) *Lacan in Contexts.* London: Verso.

Mannoni, O. (1950/1964) *Prospero and Caliban: The Psychology of Colonization.* New York: Praeger.

Marx, K. (1867) *Capital: A Critique of Political Economy*, https://www.marxists.org/archive/marx/works/1867-c1/ (accessed 29 January 2019).

Masson, J. M. (1984/1985) *The Assault on Truth: Freud's Suppression of the Seduction Theory.* Harmondsworth, UK: Penguin.

Menzies-Lyth, I. (1988) *Containing Anxiety in Institutions, Vol. I.* London: Free Association Books.

Miller, J.-A. (1968) 'Action of the structure'. In P. Hallward and K. Peden (eds) (2012), *Concept and Form, Volume 1, Selections from Cahiers pour l'Analyse.* London: Verso.

Miller, M. (1998) *Freud and the Bolsheviks: Psychoanalysis in Imperial Russia and the Soviet Union.* New Haven, CT: Yale University Press.

Millett, K. (1977) *Sexual Politics.* London: Virago.

Mitchell, J. (1974) *Psychoanalysis and Feminism*, Harmondsworth, UK: Penguin.

Monroe, A. (2005) *Interrogation Machine: Laibach and the NSK State.* Cambridge ,MA: MIT Press.

O'Connor, N. and Ryan, J. (1993) *Wild Desires and Mistaken Identities: Lesbianism and Psychoanalysis.* London: Virago.

Owens, C. (ed.) (2009) Lacan and critical psychology, annual review of critical psychology, 7, https://discourseunit.com/annual-review/7-2009/ (accessed 29 January 2019).

Owens, C. and Farrelly Quinn, S. (eds) (2017) *Lacanian Psychoanalysis with Babies, Children, and Adolescents: Further Notes on the Child.* London and New York: Routledge.

Parker, I. (1997) *Psychoanalytic Culture: Psychoanalytic Discourse in Western Society.* London: Sage.

Parker, I. (2004) *Slavoj Žižek: A Critical Introduction.* London: Pluto Press.

Parker, I. (2008) *Japan in Analysis: Cultures of the Unconscious.* London: Palgrave.

Parker, I. (2009) *Psychoanalytic Mythologies.* London: Anthem Press.

Parker, I. (2011) *Lacanian Psychoanalysis: Revolutions in Subjectivity*. London and New York: Routledge.

Parker, I. and Pavón-Cuéllar, D. (eds) (2014) *Lacan, Discourse, Event: New Psychoanalytic Approaches to Textual Indeterminacy*. London and New York: Routledge.

Parker, I. and Revelli, S. (2008) *Psychoanalytic Practice and State Regulation*. London: Karnac.

Parker, I. and Siddiqui, S. (eds) (2019) *Islamic Psychoanalysis and Psychoanalytic Islam: Cultural and Clinical Dialogues*. London and New York: Routledge.

Pavón Cuéllar, D. (2010) *From the Conscious Interior to an Exterior Unconscious: Lacan, Discourse Analysis and Social Psychology*. London: Karnac.

Pavón Cuéllar, D. (2017) *Marxism and Psychoanalysis: In or Against Psychology?* London and New York: Routledge.

Rancière, J. (1974/2011) *Althusser's Lesson*. New York: Continuum.

Reich, W. (1972) *Sex-Pol: Essays, 1929-1934*. New York: Random House.

Rogers, A. G. (1976) *The Unsayable: The Hidden Language of Trauma*. New York: Random House.

Rogers, C. (1961) *On Becoming a Person: A Therapist's View of Psychotherapy*. London: Constable.

Rose, J. (2007) *The Question of Zion* (2nd edition). Princeton, NJ: Princeton University Press.

Roudinesco, E. (1990) *Jacques Lacan & Co.: A History of Psychoanalysis in France 1925–1985*. London: Free Association Books.

Rowan, J. and Dryden, W. (eds) (1988) *Innovative Therapy in Britain*. Buckingham, UK: Open University Press.

Samuels, A. (1993) *The Political Psyche*. London and New York: Routledge.

Sartre, J.-P. (1974) *Between Existentialism and Marxism*. London: New Left Books.

Shingu, K. (1995/2004) *Being Irrational: Lacan, the Objet a, and the Golden Mean*. Tokyo: Gakuju Shoin.

Siddiqui, S. (2016) *Religion and Psychoanalysis in India: Critical Clinical Practice*. London and New York: Routledge.

Sohn-Rethel, A. (1978) *Intellectual and Manual Labour: A Critique of Epistemology*. London: Macmillan.

Stafford-Clark, D. (1967) *What Freud Really Said*. Harmondsworth, UK: Penguin.

Stavrakakis, Y. (2007) *The Lacanian Left: Psychoanalysis, Theory, Politics*. Edinburgh: Edinburgh University Press.

Stock Whitaker, D. (2000) *Using Groups to Help People*. London and New York: Routledge and Kegan Paul.

Szasz, T. (1961) *The Myth of Mental Illness*. New York: Harper & Row.

Viveiros de Castro, E. (2017) *Cannibal Metaphysics*. Minneapolis, MN: University of Minnesota Press.

Winnicott, D. W. (1974) *Playing and Reality*. Harmondsworth, UK: Penguin.

Yalom, I. D. (1989) *Love's Executioner, and Other Tales of Psychotherapy*. Harmondsworth, UK: Penguin.

Young, R. M. (1977) 'Science is social relations', *Radical Science Journal*, 5, pp. 65–129.

Young, R. M. (1994) *Mental Space*. London: Process Press.

Young, R. M. (1997) 'Psychoanalysis and psychotherapy: The grand leading the bland', http://human-nature.com/rmyoung/papers/pap101.html (accessed 29 January 2019).

Žižek, S. (1986) '"Pathological Narcissus" as a socially mandatory form of subjectivity'. In C. Lasch, *Narcisistička Kultura*. Zagreb: Naprijed.

Žižek, S. (1989) *The Sublime Object of Ideology*. London: Verso.

Žižek, S. (1993) 'Why are Laibach and NSK not fascists?' In I. Arns (ed.) (2003) *IRWINRETROPRINCIP: 1983–2003*. Frankfurt: Revolver.

INDEX

For Product Safety Concerns and Information please contact our EU
representative GPSR@taylorandfrancis.com
Taylor & Francis Verlag GmbH, Kaufingerstraße 24, 80331 München, Germany

www.ingramcontent.com/pod-product-compliance
Ingram Content Group UK Ltd.
Pitfield, Milton Keynes, MK11 3LW, UK
UKHW020202200926
475702UK00004B/569
* 9 7 8 0 3 6 7 1 4 4 3 2 6 *